100 Cases for Students of Medicine

100 Cases for Students of Medicine
Medicine, Surgery, Obstetrics and Gynaecology

Michael Gillmer MD, MRCOG

Clinical Reader in Obstetrics and Gynaecology,
Nuffield Department of Obstetrics and Gynaecology,
University of Oxford
Honorary Consultant, John Radcliffe Hospital, Oxford

David Gordon MB, BChir, MRCP

Senior Lecturer in Medicine,
St. Mary's Hospital Medical School,
London

Peter Sever MB, BChir, PhD, MRCP

Professor of Clinical Pharmacology
St. Mary's Hospital Medical School,
London

Philip Steer BSc, MB, BS, MRCOG

Lecturer in Obstetrics and Gynaecology,
St. Mary's Hospital Medical School,
London

CHURCHILL LIVINGSTONE
EDINBURGH LONDON AND NEW YORK 1979

CHURCHILL LIVINGSTONE
Medical Division of the Longman Group Limited

Distributed in the United States of America by Churchill
Livingstone Inc., 19 West 44th Street, New York,
N.Y. 10036, and by associated companies, branches and
representatives throughout the world.

First published 1979
Reprinted 1981

ISBN 0 443 01649 6

British Library Cataloguing in Publication Data
100 cases for students of medicine.
   1. Diseases — Cases, clinical reports, statistics
   I. Gillmer, Michael
   616'.09   RC66   79-41012

Printed in Hong Kong by Sing Cheong Printing Co Ltd

Preface

Practising doctors know that the most painless and efficient way to learn about disease and diagnosis is to practise. This involves taking histories, examining patients, planning investigations and discussion with colleagues. Many hang their knowledge of disease on the patients they have cared for, have seen, or discussed.

Medical students also learn in this way: but there are constraints of time, and they are often diffident about imposing themselves (as they see it) on the sick. Also, they may never meet some of the important problems that they must be capable of tackling when they graduate.

The aim of this book is to challenge, instruct and amuse the student. The reader can select the case histories at random — they are in random order — or by speciality, presenting problem, or final diagnosis: to this end, the index is in three sections. We firmly believe that the clinical skills of history taking and physical examination remain at the centre of good medical practice, and most of our cases rely on the interpretation of these rather than on special investigations.

We would like to thank many of our colleagues who have helped with advice and discussion to clarify our thoughts, but those confusions and errors that remain are our responsibility alone. We are grateful to Veronica Adams, Rene Anderson and Geraldine Bartlett for their typing.

M. Gillmer
D. Gordon
P. Sever
London, 1979   P. Steer

An author aged 43 was having a celebratory lunch with her agent in a steakhouse. Considerable quantities of burgundy had been drunk, and they had just begun their steaks when she suddenly collapsed to the floor, apparently lifeless. The agent noted that her lips and skin had turned blue, and that he could feel no pulse. He attempted mouth-to-mouth respiration (after removing her upper and lower dentures) but he failed to inflate her chest, and the blue colour became more marked.

When the ambulance men arrived they made the correct diagnosis. Although they applied the correct initial treatment, their further attempts at resuscitation failed.

1. What is the correct diagnosis?
2. What is the correct initial treatment?

This history is typical of respiratory obstruction developing acutely following aspiration of a foreign body. This can occur at any age, and with any foreign body of appropriate size that might be taken in the mouth: a child may aspirate a marble that it has been sucking: a boiled sweet given injudiciously to a baby may disappear into the larynx: an elderly person can crack their dentures and then breathe in a fragment.

Steak is notorious as a food often swallowed in chunks rather than fully masticated. A middle aged person with a complete set of false teeth is particularly likely to have difficulty in chewing, and if he or she is more or less drunk, coordination of chewing, swallowing and breathing is likely to be impaired. As the lump of steak sticks in the larynx, respiration is completely obstructed, with rapid development of cyanosis, and there is often a cardiac arrest, probably due to reflex stimulation of vagal activity.

The correct initial treatment is, as in all attempts at cardiopulmonary resuscitation, to ensure that the airway is clear: this would be the correct first manoeuvre even if our author's collapse were due to a cardiac arrest following a myocardial infarction. All that is needed is to reach over the back of the tongue and pull the lump of meat out of the larynx with the index and middle fingers of one hand. Special instruments are not necessary, although it has seriously been suggested that steakhouse waiters should be trained to lift foreign bodies out of the larynx with specially designed plastic forceps. Mouth-to-mouth respiration before clearing the airway only ensures that the foreign body is more firmly wedged in the larynx.

An English girl of 21 years was admitted to hospital after she had fainted at work. Six months previously she had complained to her family doctor of feeling tired and weak and a blood count taken at that time confirmed that she was anaemic (haemoglobin 6.0 g/dl).

The G.P. had prescribed iron tablets which the girl admitted she had taken irregularly, but a check on the tablet bottle indicated more than half the prescribed tablets had been taken.

For three weeks prior to admission she had experienced headaches for which she took analgesics and a recent development was a complaint of intermittent abdominal pain lasting a few minutes on each occasion, unrelated to food and not associated with any change in bowel habit. Her stools were well formed and brown-black in colour. Her mother had died (aged 42 years) following an operation for carcinoma of the colon.

Physical examination revealed a well nourished but pale girl with a tachycardia (100/min) and BP 100/50 mmHg. Temperature 37°C. No specific abnormalities were found in the remainder of the examination.

Investigations: Hb 7.0 g/dl. Red cells hypochromic and microcytic, WBC 6 x 10^9/l. Platelets normal. Blood urea and electrolytes normal. Chest X-ray normal. Liver function tests normal.

1. What further history is important to elicit?
2. Suggest three causes for this girl's anaemia.
3. Give five important investigations which may assist in the diagnosis of the anaemia.

Severe anaemia in a young person demands prompt and urgent investigation. The investigation suggests iron deficiency. Although dietary deficiencies and blood loss through heavy menstrual bleeding may account for significant iron deficiency anaemia, both are unlikely in view of her well nourished state and the persistence of anaemia despite treatment. Nevertheless a detailed history must be elicited concerning diet and menstrual loss. In addition, the identity and number of analgesics taken by the patient must be ascertained as aspirin and aspirin-containing compounds may cause gastrointestinal bleeding.

Her mother died at a young age from colonic cancer and further probing into the family history may bring to light additional cases of large bowel disease.

The most likely cause of this girl's anaemia is iron deficiency secondary to blood loss. Dietary factors must however be considered. Severe anaemia in a young person may be the presenting feature of an acute leukaemia, however the normal white cell count and platelets militate against this. Chronic infection, haemolysis, renal disease or occult malignancy must also be considered, but the absence of clues on physical examination and investigation make these diagnoses less likely.

Investigation should be directed towards the diagnosis of iron deficiency, determining the source of blood loss and identifying the underlying pathology.

A bone marrow aspiration with examination of cells of the haemopoeitic system and stains for iron stores is essential. A serum iron and total iron binding capacity should be done.

Stools must be examined for occult blood (positive in this case) and examination of the gastrointestinal tract by endoscopy (sigmoidoscopy and gastroscopy) and barium studies should be performed.

This girl was found to have multiple adenomatous polyps in the rectum and colon. Her mother had a similar illness and died as a result of malignancy developing in one (or several?) such polyps.

A 22 year old cocktail waitress who worked in a London nightclub first attended the hospital casualty department complaining of heavy vaginal bleeding and intermittent lower abdominal pain for one day. Her last normal period had occurred eight weeks earlier. Her menstrual cycle was normally regular with periods occurring every 28 days and lasting five days. She had been having regular intercourse over the preceding four months but had not taken contraceptive precautions because her 38 year old consort had assured her that he was sterile. Two weeks before coming to hospital she had noticed a brown discharge which had lasted 3 days. A pregnancy test performed at this time by her G.P. was positive and she requested referral for a therapeutic abortion. A week later she experienced heavy vaginal bleeding for two days associated with lower abdominal cramps and the passage of clots. She therefore assumed that she had miscarried. A slight brown vaginal discharge persisted during the following week but on the morning of admission heavy bleeding and pain recurred and she vomited three times. There were no other bowel symptoms and micturition was normal.

On examination she was rolling around the bed in pain. Her temperature was 37.7°C, pulse rate 100/min. and a blood pressure of 120/70 mmHg. There was no abnormality on inspection of the abdomen. Palpation revealed moderate suprapubic tenderness but no rebound tenderness or guarding. The bowel sounds were normal and there was no abdominal mass.

Speculum examination revealed slight bleeding through the cervix which was open and appeared to contain products of conception. On bimanual examination the uterus was tender and enlarged to eight weeks size. The cervix admitted a finger. There were no adnexal masses but there was bilateral pelvic tenderness. Investigations: Haemoglobin 10.9 g/dl, WBC 12.4 x 10^9/l, ESR 54 mm/h.

1. What further investigations would you perform on this patient?
2. What type of abortion has this patient had and what treatment would you advise?
3. Give five causes of spontaneous first trimester abortion.

This patient has an incomplete abortion complicated by sepsis. This may be due to one of several organisms including *Escherichia coli, Streptococcus faecalis,* anaerobic streptococci and *Clostridium welchii.* It is therefore important to take both aerobic and anaerobic cultures from the cervix and high vagina to establish the organism involved and its antibiotic sensitivities.

A broad spectrum antibiotic such as ampicillin or one of the cephalosporins should be given by intramuscular injection for 24 hours and then orally for 4 to 7 days. Oral metronidazole or in severe cases intramuscular clindamycin should also be given to combat anaerobic bacteria.

As soon as adequate antibiotic cover has been established the retained products of conception should be evacuated under general anaesthesia, using blunt instruments to prevent perforation of the soft uterine wall or damage to the basal endometrium from overzealous curettage.

The cause of the majority of spontaneous abortions remains unknown in clinical practice. The two most common are probably disorders of implantation and chromosomal abnormalities of the fetus. Maternal illness such as rubella, acute pyelonephritis, syphilis and untreated diabetes may also be causal. Congenital uterine anomalies and fibroids may prevent normal implantation or early embryonic development. The importance of progesterone deficiency is uncertain but may be a factor in some cases. X-rays and cytotoxic drugs may occasionally be implicated.

A 73 year old retired bank manager presented to casualty following a 'blackout' at home. His wife had seen the event and gave the following history:— the attack began with twitching of the left thumb and forefinger, which spread to involve the whole hand and then the left arm. The left foot and leg then also twitched and her husband went unconscious with groaning and foaming at the mouth. He awoke ten minutes later but his thoughts appeared confused and he could not remember the attack. He had suffered no previous attacks, was taking no drugs, and was in good general health. He smoked ten cigarettes each day. There was no history of any injury.

On examination, six hours after the attack, there were no abnormal physical signs. The patient had no memory of the attack apart from remembering some difficulty with stopping his hand from moving before he lost consciousness. His thought processes were otherwise normal.

1. What was the attack described by the patient's wife?
2. Suggest the most likely cause and two other possible causes.
3. Give six investigations that might be useful.
4. What treatment should be started?

This is a typical Jacksonian epileptic fit due to an abnormal discharge from an irritative focus in the right motor cortex.

At this age epilepsy is almost never 'idiopathic', and there is usually an identifiable structural abnormality. The most likely structural defect is a tumour, either primary or secondary. Other possible causes include scarring of the cortex due to cerebral ischaemia, or local atrophy due to many possible causes e.g. tertiary syphilis. In all elderly patients the possibility of a subdural haematoma must be borne in mind, even in the absence of any history of trauma, but it would be very unusual for this to present with a focal fit.

If computerised axial tomography (E.M.I. or C.A.T. scanning) is available this may give the diagnosis directly, and in particular may distinguish between a potentially curable meningioma and a less remediable glioma or secondary neoplasm. A skull X-ray may show calcification in a glioma, bone erosion or calcification associated with a meningioma, shift of a calcified pineal or erosion of the pituitary fossa. An electroencephalogram may confirm the anatomical site of the irritative focus. An isotope brain scan is painless and easy to perform, but does not exclude an anatomical abnormality if the appearances are normal. A lumbar puncture can be performed as there is no papilloedema but is unlikely to give useful information except in the case of cerebral syphilis. Carotid angiography may show any malignant circulation or displacement of otherwise normal vessels, and air encephalography will reveal any shift in the cerebral ventricles due to a space-occupying lesion, or dilatation of the ventricles with cerebral atrophy. Investigations should include a chest X-ray, sputum cytology and a W.R.

The patient should be started on anticonvulsant therapy at once as all epileptic fits are potentially harmful.

In this patient, carotid angiography showed a tumour in the right motor cortex, which was found at craniotomy to be a secondary deposit from a carcinoma of the bronchus that was not visible on the chest X-ray.

You are doing a locum in a busy general hospital and the casualty officer informs you that two patients have been admitted to your ward.

The first is a 16 year old boy with known insulin dependent diabetes mellitus who, one month prior to admission, had begun to feel thirsty and had developed polyuria and polydipsia and for the three days prior to admission had vomited frequently. He was taking soluble insulin 10 units each morning. On admission he was lethargic, drowsy and obviously underweight for his age and build. His breathing was laboured and there was a strong smell of acetone on his breath. His pulse was 140/min, BP 100/60 mmHg. Heart, lungs and abdomen were clinically normal.

Investigations on admission revealed: Hb 16.5 g/dl; WBC 15 x 10^9/l. Plasma sodium 144 mmol/l; potassium 5.0 mmol/l; bicarbonate less than 20 mmol/l. Blood sugar 39 mmol/l. Urea 7 mmol/l.

The second patient was a 69 year old lady who was found in a collapsed state when her daughter visited her that afternoon. She had not been well for several days. Your examination revealed clouding of consciousness, with incoherent speech and confusion. Dehydration was marked. The pulse was 130/min in atrial fibrillation and the blood pressure 110/70 mmHg.

Investigations showed: Hb 16.5 g/dl; WBC 14 x 10^9/l; Blood urea 20 mmol/l; plasma sodium 148 mmol/l; potassium 5.1 mmol/l; bicarbonate 23 mmol/l; blood sugar 59 mmol/l.

1. What is the diagnosis in each case?
2. Comment on the possible precipitating factors in the first case.
3. Outline the important differences in your management of these two cases.

The first patient was a known insulin dependent diabetic. The clinical presentation of weight loss, polyuria and polydipsia and biochemical findings indicate diabetic ketoacidosis. Loss of control of diabetes in such a patient may well indicate an intercurrent illness, particularly those of an infectious cause. However, in this case, single daily doses of soluble insulin would be highly inappropriate therapy. The duration of action of soluble insulin is 6-8 hours and adequate control of the diabetes would not be achieved with single dose soluble insulin.

In the second case, hyperglycaemia and dehydration in the absence of any major disturbance in acid-base balance suggest the diagnosis of a nonketotic, hyperosmolar diabetic precoma.

Management in both cases should be directed towards the restoration of a normal state of hydration, control of hyperglycaemia and re-establishment of a normal acid-base and electrolyte balance. Precipitating factors such as infection and myocardial infarction (in the elderly) must be treated with appropriate measures, and complications (uncontrolled atrial fibrillation in case two) controlled (digitalisation).

The important differences between the two cases are that the degree of dehydration is more severe in nonketotic hyperosmolar coma and rehydration with 0.45 per cent saline is advocated in the initial stages. Small doses of insulin are usually adequate to control hyperglycaemia.

In diabetic ketoacidosis the current procedure is to use insulin in relatively small doses, 4-10 units hourly administered as single doses or by intravenous infusion. Normal saline (initially) should be used for rehydration.

Subsequent management in both cases requires scrupulous control over fluid balance, careful assessment of electrolyte status with potassium supplements and frequent monitoring of blood glucose.

A 54 year old Irish railwayman came home drunk one night, and fell downstairs. His wife left him there until the morning, when he awoke and complained of a bad pain in his back and inability to move his legs. His wife and a friend carried him to bed, were he remained until the next day. As his legs were still immobile, he was sent to hospital.

When he was examined the neurological signs in the legs were: absent reflexes including plantar reflexes, a flaccid paralysis of all movements, absent pain and temperature sensation, but normal touch, vibration and joint position sensation. The absence of pain and temperature sensation extended onto his trunk up to a level corresponding to the T11 dermatome. The bladder was distended and the upper edge was palpated at the level of the umbilicus. He had no control over micturition. General examination showed a regular pulse, rate 96/min. There was difficulty feeling the pulse in the left arm, but it was easy to find on the right. The blood pressure in the left arm was 90/60 mmHg and in the right arm it was 160/110 mmHg. The pulses in the right groin and leg were impalpable. There was blood in the urine on microscopy.

A medical registrar made a diagnosis of polyarteritis nodosa. Soon after the patient reached the ward he complained of an excruciating pain between the shoulder blades, and dropped dead. Resuscitation was unsuccessful, and at necropsy the registrar was proved wrong.

1. Explain the neurological signs.
2. Suggest the correct diagnosis.

The only neurological functions preserved below T11 are touch, vibration and joint position sensation. These run wholly or in part in the dorsal columns of the spinal cord, dorsal to all other spinal cord tracts and neurones — including those mediating other sensations, motor functions, and bladder control — hence all the neurological abnormalities can be explained by a single lesion involving the anterior half of the spinal cord at and below T11. The symptoms were sudden in onset, so a vascular event seems likely. The anterior half to two thirds of the cord is supplied by the anterior spinal artery, so the lesion could be an acute obstruction of the anterior spinal artery.

There is also complete or partial obstruction of arteries in the left arm and right leg, and this picture of scattered arterial obstructions led the registrar to diagnose polyarteritis nodosa. Microscopic haematuria is found in polyarteritis nodosa when there is intrarenal arterial involvement, so this supported the diagnosis. However, the vessels involved in polyarteritis nodosa are usually much smaller than the major limb arteries, and arteritis involving arteries of large size is very rare and usually presents with gradual rather than acute obstructions: Takayasu's disease is an example. Pain occurred at the start and at the end of this illness, and was at one time very severe.

The correct diagnosis must be of a disease that can progress to sudden death over a few days, intermittently very painful, causing acute obstructions of major arteries to the extent that blood pressure in the two arms can be different. At postmortem, a dissecting aneurysm was found, and is compatible with all these features: the dissection extended from the arch of the aorta near the left subclavian artery to the bifurcation of the aorta and down the right common iliac artery. Haematuria is seen with dissecting aneurysm if the renal arteries are involved, and sudden death follows aortic rupture (as in this case) or retrograde dissection back to the aortic ring and pericardium.

A 38 year old housewife booked at 12 weeks in her third pregnancy when she was found to have a blood pressure of 140/90 mmHg. Her first two pregnancies, eleven and six years before, had both been complicated by pre-eclampsia and her first child had been 'small for dates'. She had no family or past history of hypertension outside pregnancy. At booking her uterine size was thought to be two weeks less than that expected from her last menstrual period, and ultrasound measurement of the fetal biparietal diameter was therefore performed. This was consistent with the estimated date of delivery calculated from the LMP. At her next antenatal visit her blood pressure was 160/100 mmHg but it was subsequently within the normal range until 28 weeks when a measurement of 140/90 mmHg was again obtained. Two weeks later this had risen to 170/100 mmHg. The uterine size at this visit was found to be equivalent to only 26 weeks. There was no oedema or proteinuria but in view of her persisting hypertension she was admitted to hospital for rest. Her blood pressure remained elevated (170/110 mmHg) and it was therefore decided to treat her with hypotensive (alphamethyldopa) and diuretic (cyclopenthiazide) drugs. After starting treatment her blood pressure fell to 140/90 mmHg but despite increasing doses of alphamethyldopa rose slowly to reach 170/110 mmHg at 35 weeks. At this stage she developed moderate proteinuria and oedema of her hands, ankles and calves. The uterine size had remained smaller than dates (equivalent to only 30 weeks gestation) with diminished liquor.

1. What investigations would you have performed in early pregnancy to determine the cause of this patient's hypertension?
2. What is the reason for using hypotensive therapy?
3. What is the most likely cause of the deterioration of her condition?
4. How would you manage the remainder of her pregnancy?

A diastolic blood pressure of 90 mmHg is not uncommon at the booking antenatal visit and is usually a reflection of the patient's anxiety. If hypertension persists it is, however, important to determine its aetiology before dismissing it as 'essential' or idiopathic'. This involves taking a detailed history with regard to renal disease, and examination of the urine for protein, granular casts and pus cells. Blood urea and uric acid, and creatinine clearance should also be measured. A thorough cardiovascular examination is also necessary to exclude the possibility of coarctation of the aorta and renal artery stenosis (suggested by a bruit overlying the renal area). Retinal changes and evidence of cardiac enlargement should also be sought as these provide an indication of the severity of the disease.

When blood pressure is very labile and especially if there are symptoms of flushing or dizziness a phaeochromocytoma should be excluded by measuring 24 hour urine VMA excretion or plasma catecholamines.

The usual fall in blood pressure which occurs in early pregnancy, meant that the true significance of this patient's hypertension was missed until the thirtieth week of pregnancy. Hypotensive therapy was used, for maternal reasons, to protect against risks of cerebral haemorrhage, left ventricular hypertrophy and malignant hypertension. It does not appear to improve the fetal prognosis nor guard against the development of pre-eclampsia. This latter complication is more common in hypertensive patients and was responsible for the deterioration of this patient's blood pressure in the third trimester and the appearance of oedema and proteinuria at 35 weeks.

Hypertension is associated with a reduced placental blood flow and this causes both intrauterine growth retardation and an increased risk of asphyxia and intrauterine death especially in labour. Fetal growth should therefore be monitored by serial ultrasound cephalometry and fetal well being by measurement of bi-weekly, plasma oestrogen or 24 hour urine oestrogen excretion, and resting cardiotocography. This latter should be performed daily if possible and may be combined with fetal movement counts. Weekly or twice weekly measurement of the plasma human placental lactogen (HPL) concentration may also be useful. The value of this intensive monitoring is that pregnancy may be allowed to continue as long as the results of the investigations remain normal, even in the presence of oligohydramnios and a uterine and fetal size smaller than expected.

Proteinuria is a finding of sinister prognostic significance and indicates the need to deliver the fetus as soon as it is considered to be mature. Respiratory distress syndrome is uncommon when hypertension complicates pregnancy or the fetus is small for dates but if there is doubt about fetal maturity the amniotic fluid lecithin-sphingomyelin ratio should be measured.

If the cervix is unfavourable or the blood pressure unstable an elective Caesarean section should be performed. If the cervix is favourable, the blood pressure well controlled, and there are no other obstetric complications then labour may be induced provided facilities for continuous fetal heart rate monitoring and pH determination are available.

A 28 year old girl presented with a six day history of intermittent abdominal pain. The pain was present most of the time but there were periods of acute exacerbation. She had recently lost several pounds in weight and felt generally unwell. Two days before admission she had felt nauseated and vomited on several occasions. Three years previously she had been admitted to a hospital in Devon with a similar illness and a diagnosis was established after investigation. She had taken prednisone tablets regularly (5 mg daily) since that time.

Physical examination revealed a thin girl with slight pallor. She was not obviously dehydrated. The temperature was 38°C, pulse rate 100/min, BP 110/80 mmHg. Examination of the rest of the cardiovascular and respiratory systems was normal. The abdomen was not distended. Generalised tenderness was elicited over the abdomen, most marked around the umbilicus and associated with guarding. There was no rebound tenderness and no palpable masses were felt. Bowel sounds were reduced in intensity.

Investigations: Hb 10.5 g/dl; WBC 15.3 x 10^9/l ESR 79 mm/h. Blood urea and electrolytes — normal; urine microscopy revealed no cells or protein and culture was negative.

1. Suggest four causes for the abdominal symptoms.
2. Which of these could be attributed to her prednisone?
3. What immediate investigations would you perform?
4. Outline your management of this case.

This girl presents with an acute abdomen and her past medical history is highly relevant. The physical signs on admission of pyrexia, abdominal tenderness and guarding suggest an inflamed or perforated viscous. It is important to remember that steroid therapy may mask some of the classical signs associated with peritonitis.

The past history of a similar illness for which she had been given steroids is highly suggestive of an inflammatory bowel disorder of which Crohn's disease is the most probable. In the absence of diarrhoea, ulcerative colitis is less likely but must be considered. The frequent occurrence of vomiting should draw your attention to the possibility of intestinal obstruction, although the absence of abdominal distension militates against this.

Other possible diagnoses include a peptic ulcer with or without perforation, acute appendicitis and acute pancreatitis. Peptic ulceration, perforation and pancreatitis can occur in association with steroid therapy.

Immediate investigations must include an examination of the stool for occult blood, an erect and supine X-ray of the abdomen for signs of gas under the diaphragm, indicative of a perforated viscus, and a serum amylase.

The locus of the pain indicates a 'midgut' distribution. Nevertheless, in view of the history and steroid treatment a gastroscopy would be indicated. Subsequently sigmoidoscopy and barium studies (meal, follow-through and enema) should be carried out.

If her condition deteriorates, a laparotomy must be performed.

At the time of his discharge (age 28) from the army, this patient had been graded 'A1'. He then went to work as a porter on the railway, and was fit and well until the age of 42, when he was admitted to hospital with a myocardial infarct. His recovery was uneventful, but the notes of that admission to hospital were lost.

At the age of 48, he presented to his general practitioner complaining of lassitude, depression, headaches, thirst, polyuria and constipation, all of which had come on gradually over about one year or more. On examination, his doctor found a rough, medium-to-low pitched, pansystolic murmur at the apex, radiating to the axilla, and a third heart sound. The railwayman was referred to a cardiologist, who noted that he was clinically anaemic, and arranged his admission to hospital for cardiac catheterisation. Investigations performed by the house physician showed:—

Hb 9.7 g/dl

Blood film — normocytic, normochromic red cells

Plasma Sodium — 137 mmol/l
       Potassium — 3.8 mmol/l
       Bicarbonate — 21 mmol/l
       Urea — 20.4 mmol/l (normal range 2.5 — 6.6)
       Creatinine — 437 μmol/l (62 — 124)
       Alkaline Phosphatase — 243 U/l (20 — 95)

Blood sugar — 4.8 mmol/l (3.0 — 5.0)

Chest X-ray — clear lung fields; slight cardiac enlargement; loss of bone density, especially at the lateral ends of both clavicles.

Abdominal X-ray — normal apart some diffuse calcification in both renal shadows.

1. What one other pair of biochemical tests would you like performed, and why?
2. What is the cause of the present symptoms?
3. What is the likely cause of the cardiac signs?

The investigations show that the patient has renal failure: the electrolytes, urea, creatinine, haemoglobin and blood film are all typical of a moderate degree of this condition. Although some bone demineralisation would be expected with renal failure of this degree, the very high alkaline phosphatase and the loss of bone density in the chest X-ray suggest that it is particularly prominent in this case. In addition, the renal calcification (nephrocalcinosis) suggests that the relative concentrations of calcium and phosphate in the blood are such that ectopic calcification can occur. The pair of investigations that is needed is measurement of calcium and inorganic phosphate concentrations in serum or plasma.

The relative concentrations of calcium and phosphate would give a clue to the state of parathyroid activity. A high calcium with a low phosphate would suggest primary hyperparathyroidism, excess parathyroid hormone (from an adenoma or carcinoma of the parathyroids, or produced ectopically, perhaps by a bronchial carcinoma) mobilising calcium from the bone by stimulating osteoclastic activity and promoting the excretion of phosphate by direct action on the renal tubules. Uncomplicated renal failure would give a low calcium, largely due to failure of absorption from the gut in the absence of active vitamin D which is synthesised in the kidney: the phosphate would tend to be high as renal excretion fails. Renal failure and hypocalcaemia would, in time, stimulate parathyroid activity and the calcium would tend to rise as it was mobilised from bone by the secondarily stimulated parathyroid hormone secretion: this is secondary hyperparathyroidism. Eventually the stimulated parathyroid overactivity might become autonomous, perhaps with development of an adenoma: this is then tertiary hyperparathyroidism. Both secondary and tertiary hyperparathyroidism produce a high serum calcium, and their association with renal failure means that the phosphate will also be high. However, primary hyperparathyroidism can lead to renal damage as a direct effect of the high calcium, and the renal damage may lead to a rise in serum phosphate: thus, the late stages of primary, secondary and tertiary hyperparathyroidism may be biochemically and clinically indistinguishable.

The presenting symptoms in this patient could perhaps all be due to renal failure, but thirst and polyuria in the absence of hyperglycaemia are strongly suggestive of hypercalcaemia: all the other presenting symptoms are also typical of a high circulating calcium. However, the cardiac signs cannot be attributed to either parathyroid or kidney disease. The murmur is that of mitral regurgitation, and a third heart sound is often heard with mitral regurgitation. His 'A1' discharge at the age of 28 makes it unlikely that the murmur was then present, or that he suffered from rheumatic fever. The clue as to cause is in the admission with myocardial infarction 6 years before his last admission: papillary muscle necrosis not uncommonly follows myocardial infarction, and papillary muscle rupture or dysfunction may lead to mitral regurgitation.

This man had hyperparathyroidism, probably tertiary. He felt much better after parathyroidectomy, but eventually died of renal failure.

A 30 year old solicitor's wife presented to the gynaecological outpatient clinic complaining of inability to conceive despite trying for three years. Her menarche occurred at the age of twelve years and she subsequently had normal regular periods. At the age of 18 years she started taking the oral contraceptive pill. Two years later she had an asymptomatic attack of gonorrhoea, detected by contact tracing, and was treated with intramuscular penicillin. When she was twenty two she stopped the pill because she had broken off her relationship with her boyfriend. However, following unpremeditated intercourse at a party, she became pregnant. This pregnancy was terminated at 10 weeks gestation, and was followed by heavy bleeding and a fever on the sixth postoperative day. She was readmitted for evacuation of retained products of conception, and discharged after three days on treatment with oral cephalexin. She was worried by current press reports on the dangers of the oral contraceptive pill and so six weeks after the operation she had an intra-uterine device fitted at a family planning clinic. However, the coil produced heavy periods, and after nine months she developed acute lower abdominal pain and the coil was removed. She therefore recommenced the contraceptive pill but discontinued this on her marriage at the age of twenty seven, hoping to become pregnant. Her periods continued to be regular over the next three years. As she failed to conceive, she started to keep a temperature chart (after reading about this in a woman's magazine) which showed a significant rise in the second half of the cycle. Initial investigations of her husband at the clinic showed he had a normal semen analysis, and a post-coital test was also normal.

1. What is the most likely cause of this woman's secondary infertility?
2. How would you confirm the diagnosis?
3. How and why could you criticise her medical management?
4. What is the likely outcome of therapy?

This patient's temperature chart suggests she is ovulating regularly and her husband appears to have normal spermatogenesis. The problem is probably a mechanical obstruction to conception caused by tubal occlusion. This must be acquired since she has already proven the lack of a congenital block by becoming pregnant, and almost certainly follows pelvic infection. The sequence of events was almost certainly as follows:

Tubal damage of a minor degree probably occurred at the time of the gonorrhoeal infection. The initial infection cannot however have caused complete tubal occlusion since she subsequently became pregnant, but the damaged tubes proved susceptible to an opportunist infection which occurred following the termination of pregnancy. This recurred after nine months due to the efeects of the intra-uterine device. Either of these two infections could have been the cause of tubal occlusion.

The diagnosis can be confirmed readily by laparoscopy and hydrotubation. This involves injecting a dye, usually methylene blue, into the uterine cavity. The fallopian tubes are simultaneously observed for the appearance of the dye from their fimbrial ends. Failure to observe the passage of dye suggests that tubal occlusion has occurred. In addition, the overall appearance of the tubes should be noted (for example, looking for hydrosalpinges, terminal clubbing, or occlusion by adhesions) since this will affect the prognosis and the type of reconstructive surgery, if any, which is recommended. Hysterosalpingography (an X-ray examination in which a radio-opaque dye is used) will appear to show tubal occlusion in twenty per cent of cases where dye can be seen to pass at laparoscopy. As a result, this investigation is now usually reserved for the delineation of the site of an occlusion already demonstrated by laparoscopy, and for the demonstration of the shape of the uterine cavity.

Since the intra-uterine contraceptive device is known to increase the incidence of pelvic inflammatory disease, its insertion in a patient with a history suggestive of this condition is strongly contraindicated. This is particularly important if a nulliparous patient wishes to have a family and can use an alternative method of contraception. For the patient who has completed her family, the coil may be acceptable but only after other methods have proved unsatisfactory. Careful supervision would then be required.

The outcome of surgery for tubal occlusion is very poor, the best result being obtained after simple division of adhesions when the tubes are otherwise undamaged. This is termed salpingolysis and has a subsequent pregnancy rate of about forty per cent. If a false ostium has to be produced (salpingostomy) the results are much worse (pregnancy rate ten per cent) because fimbrial function is abnormal. The results of tubal reanastomosis for a localised block lie between these two extremes.

A 52 year old consultant dermatologist was noted by his junior staff to be starting his Monday morning ward round later and later. He had formerly been of very punctual habits. He also sometimes failed to be present for his other ward rounds and clinics, but usually kept better time later in the week. The consultant said that he had been delayed by severe 'dyspepsia', and also revealed that his wife had recently left him. An observant registrar noted that he had lost a little weight, and pressed his chief to seek medical advice. The consultant declined to do so until one morning he was found by the registrar, vomiting blood.

1.   Give a likely diagnosis, and two other possible diagnoses.
2.   What other points in the history would be of particular importance?

The history of disturbed work and family life, weight loss, and gastrointestinal disturbance culminating in haematemesis are compatible with alcoholism. The particular difficulty with Monday morning is not unusual after a weekend of heavy drinking. It would be wrong, however, to exclue the possibility of a serious illness such as a gastrointestinal neoplasm or peptic ulcer. This would explain the weight loss, gastrointestinal symptoms and bleeding, and also the physician's unwillingness to be seen by a doctor.

When taking the history, care should be taken to ask for details of alcohol consumption. Other symptoms related to alcoholism include tremor relieved by alcohol (the 'shakes'), early morning retching, drinking bouts, and episodes of loss of memory, sometimes with impairment of thought processes and memory apparent only to the patient. A family history of alcoholism may be relevant, and alcoholics often also abuse drugs and tobacco. Enquiry should be made for details of marital and social history and the circumstances of his wife's departure. The patient is likely to be depressed, and symptoms should be enquired for directly, that is, early morning waking, fits of weeping, suicidal thoughts and so on. Other points of importance include symptoms relating to the gut — exact weight lost, dysphagia, nausea, vomiting, abdominal pain and its associated features, bleeding from the bowel and changes in bowel habit.

This man was an alcoholic. He was unable to alter his habits and resigned his post shortly before dying from bleeding oesophageal varices.

12

A 23 year old boy was admitted to hospital after breaking his leg in a game of rugby. On admission to Casualty, he was in great pain and clinical examination revealed a fracture of the shaft of the right tibia, which on subsequent X-ray was shown to be displaced. No other injury had been sustained.

Under a general anaesthetic the fracture was reduced and immobilised in an above knee plaster of paris cast.

During the ensuing 36 hours his general condition was satisfactory. He was alert and sitting up in bed. The following evening it was noted by the nursing staff that he was a little confused. His pulse was regular, 100/min; BP 110/70 mmHg, respiratory rate 30/min.

He apparently settled down for the night and was noted to be sleeping 'normally' by the night staff. At 6 a.m. the following morning, he was found dead in his bed.

1. How do you account for the confusion noted on the evening prior to his demise?
2. What investigations should have been carried out?
3. What was the cause of death?

Deterioration in the level of consciousness after a major injury should alert the physician to the possibility of intracranial injury or fat embolism syndrome. The former is less likely in this case as there was no history of head injury. Nevertheless, a full neurological examination should have been performed when he was noted to be confused, with attention devoted to the identification of lateralising signs which could indicate an extradural haemorrhage.

Fat embolism occurs following trauma, particularly that involving long bones and usually within 48 hours of the initial injury. Characteristically this phenomenon is associated with the development of petechial haemorrhages in the skin due to fat emboli in the microcirculation. The presentation is that of a progressive respiratory embarrassment with a falling arterial Po_2 and cerebral anexia. Chest pain is uncommon.

Measurement of arterial blood gases would have demonstrated anoxia at the time of confusion and suggested the diagnosis. The associated hyperventilation should have alerted the medical staff to the probability of an underlying pulmonary problem. Pulmonary emboli would be unusual so soon after the accident.

The chest X-ray is usually normal with fat emboli, but urine to which osmic acid is added turns black due to staining of the fat.

Anoxia requires the prompt administration of oxygen. If little improvement occurs in the arterial Po_2 ventilation is mandatory.

A 32 year old primigravid candle maker had been married for 5 years. For one year after her marriage she had used oral contraception but subsequently stopped in order to have a child. After three years of infertility she and her husband had been investigated and both were found to be normal. Six months after the investigations had been completed she conceived.

She first attended the antenatal clinic when 16 weeks pregnant. The uterine size was compatible with the duration of the pregnancy calculated from the last menstrual period and she appeared healthy. Her pregnancy progressed normally and the fetal lie remained longitudinal with a cephalic presentation from the thirtieth week. Pelvic assessment at 36 weeks revealed a favourable pelvic shape and adequate dimensions. Twelve days after the expected date of delivery she complained of reduced fetal movements.

On examination the fetal lie was longitudinal, the head was engaged and the fetal and uterine size corresponded to term. Her blood pressure was 130/80 mmHg. Her total weight gain since booking was 9.5 kg and there was neither oedema nor any abnormality on urine analysis. Vaginal examination revealed that the fetal head was at the level of the ischial spines, the cervix was soft, central, 3 centimetres dilated, and approximately 80 per cent effaced. Because of her complaint of reduced fetal movements resting cardiotocography was performed to assess fetal well being and this was normal. In view of the postmaturity, her age and previous infertility it was however decided to induce labour by simultaneous low amniotomy and intravenous oxytocin infusion.

At the time of rupturing the membranes the amniotic fluid was noted to be slightly meconium stained and a fetal scalp electrode was applied. The continuous fetal heart rate trace was normal with a baseline rate of approximately 130 beats per minute and baseline variability of ± 5 beats per minute. Four hours later she was in established labour and fifteen minutes after insertion of an epidural catheter the fetal heart rate rose to 170 beats per minute. The baseline variability was reduced and there were decelerations of approximately 50 beats per minute lasting about 30 seconds with their nadir about 20 seconds after each contraction.

1. What is the most likely cause of this fetal heart rate pattern?
2. What action would you take?

This patient has almost certainly developed hypotension caused by the epidural anaesthetic. This results in diminished placental perfusion and may cause fetal distress. In addition placental function may become impaired after term leading to intrauterine asphyxia and this has been said to account for the increased perinatal mortality observed in patients whose pregnancies continue after 42 weeks. Mechanical factors such as the large fetal size and poor moulding of the more ossified skull are probably also important. The presence of meconium in the amniotic fluid is associated with an increased incidence of fetal distress and may be indicative of pre-existing fetal stress in the present case.

It is important to ensure that the patient is lying on her side to prevent supine hypotension, to check her blood pressure and if this is low and there is no contraindication (e.g. cardiac disease), to give one litre of normal saline by rapid intravenous infusion.

The oxytocin infusion rate should be checked in case a large bolus of oxytocin has been administered inadvertently. If the fetal heart pattern has not returned to normal within 20-30 minutes of correcting the hypotension a fetal scalp blood sample should be taken, if the pH is less than 7.25 then delivery should be expedited, if necessary, by means of Caesarean section. Other causes of sudden fetal distress in labour include cord prolapse and concealed *abruptio placentae* and these complications should be considered if correction of the hypotension does not restore the fetal heart rate trace to normal.

A 51 year old bus driver complained to his workmates that the previous week, following a heavy night's frost, he was aware of a 'rheumatic pain' in his left shoulder and arm when walking to the bus depot. He was advised to rub liniment on his shoulder and after a further week the pain disappeared.

One month later he was trying to start his car with a starting handle and developed acute breathlessness with a dull ache in the chest which remained for one hour until he was taken to the nearest hospital.

On arrival he was pale, sweating profusely and in pain. His pulse was 100/min, regular; BP 100/70 mmHg; JVP not elevated. No abnormalities were found in the cardiovascular system, but on auscultation of the chest widespread crepitations were audible. Examination of the abdomen and c.n.s. revealed no abnormalities.

1. What was the correct diagnosis for the shoulder pain, and give two precipitating causes.
2. What was the diagnosis on arrival at the hospital? State the complication present at this time.
3. Outline your immediate therapy.

The pain in the shoulder and arm was almost certainly that of angina. Angina 'pectoris' may occur in its classical form as a central tight chest pain radiating to the shoulders, arms or neck and jaw, but occasionally presents with pain solely at the site of radiation. It is most commonly precipitated by exertion and many patients are aware of the effect of cold weather in producing their symptoms as in this case.

The diagnosis on arrival at hospital was that of a myocardial infarction, highly probable in view of the previous history. Nevertheless, other possibilities such as a dissecting aneurysm should be borne in mind. The breathlessness and the presence of crepitations in the lung fields suggests pulmonary oedema.

The immediate treatment consists of pain relief with morphine or heroin; oxygen by mask (maximum concentration) and intravenous frusemide to relieve the pulmonary congestion. Digitalisation may be subsequently required.

The patient was a 45 year old Iranian tourist, who was writhing in pain and clutching his right side. The history was obtained with difficulty through an interpreter. It appeared that he had been awoken in the night by excruciating pain in the right loin which had radiated down to the right testicle.

He had suffered an attack of pain two years previously: this pain had been identical in every respect to the present episode except that it had been on the left, and the pain had persisted until an operation involving a 'basket' had been performed. No signs of any operation scars could be seen on examination. Since his twenties he had suffered from epigastric pain after food, which he treated by drinking five pints of milk each day, as well as taking quantities of antacid medicines.

Investigations showed: plasma calcium 2.71 mmol/l (normal 2.25-2.62), albumin 45 g/l (35-50), alkaline phosphatase 84 iu (30-115), creatinine 132 μmol/l (60-120). X-ray of the hands showed normal bones with no subperiosteal erosions and normal terminal phalanges.

1. What is the likely cause of the pain?
2. What is the relevance of the epigastric pain, and of the X-ray of the hands?

Severe pain radiating from loin to groin, sometimes also to the testis or labia, is typical of ureteric colic and is usually due to obstruction of the ureter by stone. As with this patient, the victim rolls around in agony, unable to find a position that gives any relief until adequate analgesia has been given. The past history of a similar episode supports this diagnosis, and it sounds as though the stone on the left was snared in a Dormia basket introduced into the ureter at cystoscopy — hence the lack of operation scars.

In any patient with calculi in the urinary tract the question must be asked: why have they formed? If a remediable cause is missed, needless pain and risk may follow from further stones. Unfortunately, a remediable cause — infection; stasis; pathological aminoaciduria and so on — is unusual. Often, the only abnormality on investigation is a tendency for the renal excretion of calcium to be high for no apparent reason, so-called idiopathic hypercalciuria. Hypercalcaemia, which is usually accompanied by hypercalciuria, is much less common, but is present in this patient and cannot be explained by a high plasma albumin concentration. An obvious derangement of normal physiology that can cause hypercalcaemia is oversecretion of parathyroid hormone (hyperparathyroidism) with excessive mobilisation of calcium from bone. This is accompanied by a rise in alkaline phosphatase and evidence of bone erosion on X-ray: in the hands the changes are typically subperiosteal erosions in the phalanges, with loss of definition of the tips of the terminal phalanges. There is no evidence in this man that the excess circulating calcium is from bone (the alkaline phosphatase and the hand X-rays are normal) although there is evidence, in the slightly raised plasma creatinine, of impaired renal function, which may be found in hypercalcaemia of any cause.

If the excess plasma calcium is not from bone then maybe excess calcium is being absorbed from the gut. This could be due either to vitamin D poisoning or to unusually high dietary calcium. This man's diet is certainly excessive in calcium, and he is an example of the milk-alkali syndrome: hypercalcaemia (and other changes) due to excessive consumption of milk and alkalis taken as a treatment for dyspepsia. However, it is not certain to what extent renal stones occur because of the milk-alkali syndrome and to what extent any association is only chance. The milk-alkali syndrome has become rare now that treatments for peptic ulcer are available that are more effective than antacids.

An airline administrator aged 42 had never married and only had occasional boyfriends. Coitus was therefore infrequent and although she never used any contraception, she had only become pregnant once, at the age of 25. This pregnancy was terminated at ten weeks gestation. Her periods were always regular, with bleeding for 2-3 days every 28. She had never had any dysmenorrhoea, intermenstrual or postcoital bleeding.

About three weeks before her appearance in the outpatient clinic, she had experienced sudden onset of lower abdominal pain which was worst in the right iliac fossa but also spread across to the midline. Initially the pain was colicky and she vomited once, but after a few hours it settled to a dull ache. One week later she had a normal period. After a further week the pain recurred. She consulted her general practitioner who felt a lower abdominal mass and referred her to the gynaecology clinic.

On examination there was an eighteen week cystic swelling arising out of the pelvis. The uterus, which was of normal size and retroverted, was easily palpable separate from the swelling.

1. What was the swelling most likely to be?
2. What was the cause of the abdominal pain?
3. Why had the patient not previously noticed such a large swelling?
4. What was the treatment?

The swelling was most likely to be an ovarian cyst. Uterine fibromyomata can also give rise to large asymptomatic pelvic swellings, but they are more likely to cause symptoms such as menorrhagia and dysmenorrhoea. In addition, for a fibroid of eighteen weeks size to be palpable separate from the uterus would mean that it was pedunculated, and it is most unlikely that a pedunculated fibroid would have reached this size without causing symptoms. Ovarian cysts can cause pain of sudden onset because of rupture, torsion or haemorrhage. Rupture is usually followed by the signs of peritoneal irritation, with collapse, vomiting and abdominal pain. With torsion or haemorrhage into the cyst the symptoms may in contrast be mild and intermittent. It is not possible to distinguish these latter two conditions on the history and physical examination alone.

The gradual increase in abdominal girth produced by ovarian cysts or fibroids developing in middle age is often attributed by the patient to 'middle aged spread'.

Management of ovarian tumours is always by surgical removal. The risk of malignancy varies with age. Those occurring in children are usually malignant, but otherwise the risk is said to be 20 per cent before the menopause and 50 per cent after. The tumour is more likely to be malignant if it is fixed, solid, nodular and irregular, or bilateral. Provided the tumour seems benign there is a strong case for safeguarding ovarian function in young women by dissecting out the tumour and conserving as much ovary as possible. However, in the case described above, the patient was approaching the menopause and had no wish for a family. It was therefore decided to remove the whole ovary as a precautionary measure. If there is any suggestion of malignancy, the correct management in all cases is bilateral oöphorectomy and total hysterectomy.

A 26 year old student complained of abdominal pain and fullness. The pain was mild, constant and localised to the epigastrium. Although the pain was not related to food, the feeling of fullness was made much worse by a meal. He had lost about half a stone in weight. There were no other symptoms on direct questioning. He did not drink alcohol or smoke. He had been born in Hong Kong of Chinese parents and had lived in London since he arrived from Asia two years previously.

On examination there was a mass occupying the upper part of the abdomen extending to below the umbilicus, the edge of the mass being smooth and the surface rounded. It was not possible to get between the mass and the right costal margin. A systolic bruit could be heard over the mass. There was dullness to percussion and absent breath sounds at the right base posteriorly.

1. What is the most likely diagnosis? Does this explain the signs in the chest?
2. Give four relevant investigations.
3. What treatments are available?

In a young Chinaman an hepatoma is the most likely cause of these symptoms and signs. The mass is related to the liver, as can be told from the inability to get between the mass and the right costal margin. Other causes of a greatly enlarged liver, such as secondary carcinoma, reticulosis or infection (such as an abscess) are all very much less common in young Chinese, as are the other primary tumours arising in the liver, cholangiocarcinoma or haemangioblastoma.

The signs in the chest may be due to upward displacement of the diaphragm by tumour or to a pleural effusion such as might follow infiltration of the pleura with neoplasm.

A chest X-ray will confirm which of these has occurred, and a plain abdominal X-ray might show the size of the tumour and possibly calcification in its substance. Biochemical liver function tests may show evidence of hepatocellular damage (elevation of the aminotransferases) and of obstruction of biliary passages (elevated alkaline phosphatase). An isotope liver scan should be done; a scan using technetium colloid will show an hepatoma as a filling defect, but using selenomethionine the hepatoma will take up the isotope. If exact anatomical localisation of the tumour is needed, for example before any surgery, then a coeliac axis angiogram will show which lobe or lobes of the liver are involved. Definite histology could be obtained by liver biopsy but this is a potentially dangerous procedure. A less invasive method is measurement of the serum alpha-fetoprotein, which may show elevated levels if the diagnosis of hepatoma is correct. The Australia (hepatitis B) antigen is commonly found in Chinese and in patients with hepatoma: a causal relationship has been proposed.

If the tumour is confined to one lobe, then hemihepatectomy may be surgically possible. If both lobes are affected liver transplantation (in a specialist unit) offers the only slim hope. Radiotherapy and chemotherapy are usually ineffective.

The tumour involved both lobes of the liver; the patient died soon after returning to Hong Kong.

18

A 25 year old medical student presented to her family practitioner with a complaint of frequent and severe headaches. For several years she had suffered from headaches at approximately two monthly intervals and on each occasion they were associated with nausea, vomiting and prostration. Four months before her present consultation, she had started taking oral contraceptives. The headaches increased in frequency and became more severe. She stated that she knew when her headache was about to begin because she was aware of flashing stars in her eyes which impaired her vision, and this was invariably worse in the left eye. About 15 minutes later a severe headache would develop, which would last for several hours and would be associated with vomiting. Simple analgesics were seldom effective. Her mother also complained of frequent headaches although apparently not as severe or frequent.

On examination, the only abnormality detected was a blood pressure of 160/100 mmHg.

1. Discuss the possible causes of this girl's headaches.
2. To what might their recent deterioration be attributable?
3. How would you manage the problem?

The long history of headaches, their periodicity and the description of the more recent attacks with a visual aura followed by headache, nausea and vomiting suggest a diagnosis of migraine. The positive family history is also relevant.

The length of the history militates against an intracranial lesion. Neurological signs are characteristically absent, however, during the aura, focal abnormalities may be elicited in some patients with migraine, e.g. visual field defects (hemianopia) or transient unilateral sensory or motor signs in the limbs.

The worsening of attacks and their increase in frequency following the oral contraceptive are not uncommon observations and the finding of a raised blood pressure may also be relevant as this can also be related to the pill. Although early morning headaches occur in some hypertensive subjects they are usually associated with higher pressures than those recorded in this girl. Nevertheless, migraine headaches are often more severe in the hypertensive patient.

In the management of this girl, the initial policy would be to withdraw the oral contraceptive and to recommend an alternative method of contraception. Her blood pressure should be taken on several subsequent occasions and if it remained elevated, appropriate investigations should be performed to exclude an underlying cause for her hypertension (urine microscopy, renal function studies, intravenous pyelogram, urinary VMA, etc.).

For the headaches, in the acute attack, ergotamine with or without caffeine is an effective treatment and antiemetics may also be prescribed. Should the attacks continue to occur at frequent intervals, a prophylactic agent such as clonidine would be appropriate.

A Czech clerk was forced to leave Czechoslovakia with her engineer husband during the Russian invasion. Her first pregnancy proceeded normally until thirty eight weeks gestation when her blood pressure rose to 150/90 mmHg, and she developed slight finger oedema. She was admitted for rest and observation. An ultrasound scan to check foetal growth revealed a biparietal diameter of 9.48 cm and a breech presentation. Over the next four days, her blood pressure settled to 120/70 mmHg, urine analysis was normal, and her haemoglobin was 12.6 g/dl. Twenty four hour total urinary oestrogen excretion was 115 mmol (normal). Continuous fetal heart rate monitoring for half an hour daily showed a normal reactive pattern.

1. What are the dangers of vaginal breech delivery?
2. What further investigation would you like to have performed before contemplating vaginal delivery in this patient?
3. What mode of delivery do you consider to be correct for this patient?

The main dangers of vaginal breech delivery are fetal distress due to dysfunctional labour (which occurs frequently because the ill-fitting presenting part is inefficient as a cervical dilator), an increase in the incidence of fetal asphyxia during the second stage (due to early cord occlusion) and trauma, due to lack of moulding of the aftercoming head and excessive traction during delivery. Breech presentation is associated with prematurity (30 per cent), fetal abnormality (25 per cent) and misdiagnosis (as in this case the maxim 'a head which is deeply engaged may not be there at all' is worth remembering). All these factors result in a perinatal mortality which is three times higher for breeches than for vertex delivery. It is normal to perform X-ray pelvimetry before contemplating a vaginal breech delivery. This is because it is particularly important to exclude cephalopelvic disproportion. In breech delivery the largest part of the fetus comes last, and in the event of obstruction the baby would certainly be dead or damaged before delivery could be achieved. Provided a clinical assessment of the pelvic outlet is normal, erect lateral pelvimetry is usually adequate. If there is any suggestion that the subpubic arch is narrow or the ischial spines prominent (as they were in this case) a full pelvimetry should be performed including antero-posterior views. The results in this case were:

Antero-posterior diameters:	Inlet 12.4 cm.
(From the lateral film)	Midcavity 14.0 cm.
	Outlet 11.7 cm.
Transverse diameters:	Brim 13.0 cm.
(From the A.P. film)	Interspinous 10.0 cm.
	Intertuberous 11.7 cm.

Available outlet (Outlet minus the waste space of Morris)   10.2 cm.

The X-rays showed that the pelvis was gynecoid, with moderate side wall convergence but normal spines, sacrum and sacro-iliac notches.

Some obstetricians consider that all cases of breech presentation should be delivered by Caesarean section. Most, however, will allow vaginal delivery provided the pelvimetry is normal and there are no additional complicating factors such as pre-eclampsia. In addition, some advocate induction of labour at 39 weeks gestation so that the baby is a little smaller and its head more easily moulded at delivery. The progress of labour is also important and in the event of slow progress, Caesarean section should be resorted to without delay.

In the present case, spontaneous rupture of membranes occurred at 39 weeks gestation and as her hypertension had settled it was decided to let the labour continue.

The first stage lasted 7 hours, and the pH of a fetal blood sample at full dilatation was 7.33 (normal). Assisted breech delivery was performed with Simpson's forceps to the aftercoming head. The infant was a male with an Apgar score of 9 at one minute and 10 at five minutes. Mother and baby subsequently did well.

This lady, who was aged 52, was noted for complaining. She was married, had two children, smoked 30 cigarettes each day, and worked in a canteen. She had never been ill until she suffered a pulmonary embolus. When she was about to be tailed off her warfarin, three months after the embolism, she began to complain of pain. This pain was sometimes in one place, and sometimes in another: it was often at one site for days on end. The usual places were high in her back, near the right iliac crest, in the lumbar spine radiating to the left groin, and in her head. There were never any abnormal physical signs apart from slight tenderness at each site of pain. Although she said the pain was very severe, she seemed able to get to the outpatient clinic with little effort: this was taken as evidence that her complaints were neurotic, but in retrospect it should have been regarded as a sign of great stoicism.

One year after the pulmonary embolus, a new registrar decided to review the problem. She took a careful history, and concluded that the most frequent site for pain was in the region of the fourth thoracic vertebra. There were no new signs on examination, but there was a slight protein precipitate on testing the urine with salicylsulphonic acid. She arranged an X-ray of the painful area which showed that one pedicle of T4 was absent, although it could be seen on an overpenetrated chest X-ray from a year before. Other investigations showed:—

Hb	10.4 g/dl
WBC	9.5 x 10⁹/1
Blood film	Occasional plasma cells seen
ESR	127 mm/h
Plasma urea	9.3 mmol/l (normal 2.5-6.6 mmol/l)

1. Suggest two possible diagnoses.
2. Is the pulmonary embolus relevant?
3. Give at least six useful investigations.

Total destruction of any area of bone must be by infection or neoplasm. Infection could be with pyogenic organisms or tuberculosis, and in particular tuberculosis can obliterate an area of bone with no signs of inflammatory reaction in the surrounding tissues or bones. However, spinal tuberculosis is usually in the vertebral bodies rather than posteriorly in the pedicles, and the multiple foci of pain suggest a multi-focal bone lesion, which would be rather unusual for bone tuberculosis. A neoplastic process could be secondary carcinoma — say, from a clinically undetectable primary in breast or bronchus — or a disease that tends to attack bone in the first instance, myeloma. The anaemia and high ESR would fit with any of these diagnoses, and the high ESR is especially likely in tuberculosis or myeloma. A slightly elevated blood urea could be due to the renal impairment often seen with myeloma, and also pointing to this diagnosis are the plasma cells in the blood film and the proteinuria. Bone pain in myeloma is often very severe.

An unexplained pulmonary embolus should always arouse suspicions. Did it follow an episode that the patient has forgotten when she took to her bed because of the pain? Is there a pelvic neoplasm obstructing venous flow? Does she have a neoplasm causing hypercoagulability, perhaps of pancreas or bronchus?

Further investigation can begin with a simple ward test. Does the urine protein show the characteristics of Bence-Jones protein, precipitating on warming and redissolving on boiling? Immunoelectrophoresis of urine protein will show which light chain is present if it is Bence-Jones protein. Plasma protein electrophoresis will show if there is a monoclonal band, and if it is present, plasma protein immunoelectrophoresis will be needed to classify the immunoglobulin in the monoclonal band.

Another simple ward investigation is a Mantoux test for tuberculin sensitivity, and a chest X-ray should be taken to look for active tuberculosis. The other X-rays needed are a full skeletal survey for other bone lesions, inflammatory or neoplastic. Bone marrow should be examined in case it has been replaced by neoplastic plasma cells ('myeloma cells'). Other useful tests would be a serum or plasma calcium (often high in myeloma) and chemical tests of renal function, such as serum creatinine.

The diagnosis in this patient was indeed myeloma, and she died after about one year of treatment with steroids and melphelan.

The 26 year old nulliparous wife of a pharmacist had suffered from 'wind' for some months, for which her husband had given her antacids. On Christmas Day, in the evening, she was taken ill with severe epigastric pain. The pain, which came on over five minutes, was at its most severe for one hour, then gradually improved until by the next morning the patient felt only a slight soreness. The pain was central in the epigastrium, radiating to the tip of the right scapula. The patient moved about the bed in an effort to get comfortable, and gained only slight relief from a hot-water bottle held against the abdomen. She was nauseated, and vomited once. She said that she had suffered a similar but much less severe attack some months before, while staying with a friend. No other history of possible relevance could be found. Her only other medication was an oral contraceptive, which she had taken regularly.

On examination, there was no fever. Examination of the abdomen, including rectal examination, was normal apart from marked epigastric and right upper quadrant tenderness, with some guarding.

1. What is the most likely diagnosis?
2. Is an emergency laparatomy indicated?
3. What tests should be performed?

All the features of the history and examination are consistent with a diagnosis of pain due to gall-stones. The history of 'wind' points to this diagnosis, although flatulent dyspepsia alone is by no means always associated with disease of the gall bladder. Gall-stone colic is often precipitated by large fatty meals, such as are taken at Christmas, but dietary and alcoholic excesses can also cause an acute gastritis, although the pain is not usually as severe as that described, and more vomiting would be likely. A peptic ulcer is a possible but unlikely diagnosis in the absence of a history of pain occurring regularly after food. Acute pancreatitis can cause pain of similar severity and radiation, but the victim usually remains still, often sitting forward in bed. Gall-stones are not uncommon in young women.

There is no need for an emergency laparotomy if there is no evidence of peritonitis or of a condition likely to lead to peritonitis. For example, absence of fever and of lower abdominal pain make appendicitis very unlikely. However, a laparotomy is not a very risky procedure in the young and fit, and in the event of any doubt about the diagnosis, expert surgical advice should be sought.

The urine should be tested for bile pigments as these may be excreted in increased amounts in gall-stone colic. They are also excreted during attacks of pancreatitis, and a serum amylase may help to distinguish the two. A plain X-ray of the abdomen will show about 10 per cent of gall-stones, and if this is normal an oral cholecystogram should follow.

The cholecystogram showed multiple small stones. After cholecystectomy, the patient suffered no more attacks of pain, and was free of 'wind'.

A 55 year old lady was referred to a medical clinic. She had been ill for several years complaining of breathlessness on exertion, acute pain and discolouration of the hands in cold weather and latterly difficulty in swallowing her food.

Two years previously a cardiologist had examined her and found no evidence of cardiac disease.

A physical examination was carried out by a student in the clinic. He reported to the consultant the following abnormal physical signs: a bluish discolouration and tapering of the fingers, tachypnoea and basal crepitations in the chest. He attributed the symptoms and signs in the hands to Raynaud's phenomenon, but could not account for the respiratory signs.

1. Was the diagnosis of Raynaud's correct, and what further important physical signs in the hands should be sought?
2. How do you account for the chest symptoms and signs? Give three appropriate investigations of the respiratory system.
3. Why does the patient complain of dysphagia?

Painful fingers associated with colour change on exposure to cold as described in this patient are characteristic of Raynaud's phenomenon. This condition, which reflects an impairment in the blood supply to the extremities may occur as an isolated phenomenon (Raynaud's disease) or may occur in association with other conditions ('connective tissue diseases', the presence of a cervical rib, local trauma or, as is becoming increasingly recognised, drug induced-by ß-blocking drugs).

In this particular case the coexistence of chest symptoms and signs suggests a multisystem disease as scleroderma. In this condition Raynaud's is associated with pathological changes in the skin and subcutaneous tissues producing tethering of the former to underlying tissues and the loss of skin elasticity. This is occasionally associated with subcutaneous calcification. It is not exclusively confined to the extremities and may be evident in the face and neck.

The chest symptoms and signs result from a progressive pulmonary fibrosis that occurs in many patients with scleroderma. The fine crackling crepitations are quite different on auscultation from those present in, for example, pulmonary oedema, and are due to the opening and closing of thickened alveolar walls during respiration. Lung fibrosis produces a restrictive pulmonary deficit with impairment of the ventilation-perfusion ratio. In addition tests of gas transfer are also abnormal. Thus in addition to a chest X-ray which may show increased basal shadowing, tests of pulmonary function such as FEV1/FVC (both reduced); arterial blood gases (decreased Po_2, decreased Pco_2) and diffusion capacity for carbon monoxide (reduced) should be performed.

Dysphagia when associated with scleroderma is due to the infiltration of the oesophageal wall with fibrous tissue leading to impaired peristalsis of the oesophagus during swallowing.

A 33 year old Malaysian women had had her first child at the age of 19. It had been born normally at term but had only weighed 2.95 kg. For the next 14 years she was involuntarily infertile but eventually conceived without medical aid and first attended the antenatal clinic when 11 weeks pregnant. Her uterine size was compatible with that expected from the date of her last menstrual period. She attended the antenatal clinic regularly and no complication was detected until 32 weeks when the fetal lie was noted to be transverse. As no contraindication to external cephalic version existed the fetal lie was gently corrected to longitudinal.

She was subsequently seen at weekly intervals but at each visit the fetal lie was transverse. Further attempts at version were made at 33 and 34 weeks but their success was only temporary.

1. What investigations would you perform to determine the cause of this patient's unstable lie?
2. What complications may arise as a result of a persistent transverse lie and how can they be avoided?
3. List the contraindications to external cephalic version.

The lax abdominal and uterine wall of the multiparous patient is said to be the commonest cause of an unstable lie but this diagnosis can only be made by exclusion of other causes. Ultrasound scanning is the most valuable diagnostic tool in this condition as it enables most causes to be recognised including multiple pregnancy, placenta praevia, fibroids, hydrocephalus, polyhydramnios and pelvic tumours (e.g. an ovarian cyst or cervical fibroid). With a plain abdominal X-ray only multiple pregnancy and hydrocephalus can usually be diagnosed but as fetal bony abnormalities may also be recognised an X-ray should always be performed when an unstable lie occurs in association with polyhydramnios.

If placenta praevia is excluded a vaginal examination should always be performed to exclude a pelvic tumour or contracture.

Patients with an unstable lie are at increased risk of cord prolapse when the membranes rupture spontaneously. Prolapse of an arm may also occur at this time and if the patient is in labour this may lead to an impacted shoulder presentation or even uterine rupture if preventive action is not taken. It is for this reason that all patients with an unstable lie should be admitted to hospital after the thirty-seventh week of pregnancy and if there is no contraindication to vaginal delivery many obstetricians correct the fetal lie each day. If labour has not commenced at term the lie should be corrected and an intravenous syntocinon infusion started if the head will stay over the pelvic brim. The membranes should be ruptured once contractions have commenced to encourage the head to descend into the pelvis. If this is not possible a Caesarean section should be performed.

If an unstable lie occurs in a subsequent pregnancy a uterine anomaly (such as bicornuate uterus) should be excluded by an interval hysterogram.

Contraindications to external cephalic version include a uterine scar, fibroids, a uterine anomaly, hypertension (because of the risk of placental abruption), multiple pregnancy, placenta praevia and a history of antepartum haemorrhage. It should also be avoided in rhesus negative patients because of the fetomaternal transfusion which it may cause.

A 60 year old man was recovering from a myocardial infarct in hospital. Five days after transfer from the coronary care unit to a general ward, he woke up one morning with severe pain in his left leg. The house physician was called and made the following notes: 'complained of pain in left leg, no obvious swelling or calf tenderness; pulse 125/min irregular; BP 120/80 mmHg; no cardiac failure'. An e.c.g. showed atrial fibrillation and the signs of a resolving posterior infarct.

1. What important observations were not recorded by the houseman?
2. Give two possible causes for the pain in the leg.
   (The pain became progressively worse over the next two hours.)
3. What would be your further management of this case and suggest appropriate treatment.

The vital observations in this case should have been the colour and temperature of the left leg compared with the right leg and the presence or absence of the femoral, popliteal and pedal pulses. A pale, cold pulseless leg indicates arterial embolism which may follow the myocardial infarct. The parent thrombus may form on an area of damaged endocardium or particularly if an arrythmia is present, in the left atrium. Venous thromboses commonly occur after myocardial infarction particularly if patients have been confined to bed for a prolonged period.

A surgical opinion is mandatory in this case. Anticoagulants have little place in the management of arterial emboli, but may prevent further thrombus formation. Following radiographic visualisation of the site and extension of the embolus by arteriography, arteriotomy and embolectomy would be the appropriate treatment.

25

A 25 year old medical secretary was in excellent health apart from episodes of faintness. These could come on without warning at any time of day, might last from a few seconds to about five minutes, and could occur from once a week (or less) to three or four times each day. One day she mentioned to a medical registrar who was at hand that she felt faint. He felt her pulse and found it to be indistinct, regular, and 180 beats per minute. An e.c.g. after the faintness had passed showed that the rate was then 70/min, and regular. The e.c.g. was normal in most respects, but the P-R interval was very short, and, instead of a sharp and clearly demarcated start to the QRS complexes, there was a gradual upward slur in the trace from the isoelectric line into the R wave.

1. What is the diagnosis?
2. What is the cause of the episodes of faintness?

This is the Wolff-Parkinson-White syndrome. The diagnosis is made from the electrocardiogram, which shows (as in this case), a shortened P-R interval with a slur, the delta wave, into the QRS complex. This e.c.g. picture is due to premature excitation of part of the ventricles, although the P-S interval is near normal, showing that the rate of conduction of atrial impulses to at least part of the ventricles is normal. It is not certain whether the abnormally rapid atrioventricular conduction is through abnormal tissues in the AV node or the bundle of His, or through a completely separate pathway.

The important clinical feature of the Wolff-Parkinson-White syndrome is the tendency to paroxysms of supraventricular tachycardia. This was the cause of the episode of faintness in this patient. She was much improved by propranolol 40 mg b.d., but still suffers very occasional brief runs of tachycardia.

A German woman of 58 years was referred to the gynaecology clinic by her GP because she complained of post coital bleeding. This had occurred on three occasions during the preceding month and was associated with an offensive but non-irritant vaginal discharge. It was the only vaginal bleeding the patient had experienced since the menopause eight years earlier. Just prior to referral she had also developed a urinary infection but this had cleared after antibiotic therapy. She was also troubled by minor dyspeptic symptoms but her appetite was excellent and her weight steady.

She had had 'gonorrhoea' at the age of 26 and had subsequently failed to conceive although she had never used contraception. Her first husband had died and she had been separated from her second husband for six years. During this time she had only had sexual intercourse on a few occasions. On examination she was found to be obese but otherwise fit and there was no abnormality of her chest or abdomen. The vulva was normal apart from slight atrophic changes. Speculum examination revealed a yellow vaginal discharge and a large ulcerated area on the anterior lip of the cervix. This was extremely friable and bled when a cervical smear was taken. On bimanual examination it was apparent that the ulcer was firm and indurated. The uterus appeared to be normal in size, anteverted and mobile. There were no pelvic masses nor any thickening in the vaginal fornices.

1. What is the most likely diagnosis?
2. What further investigations would you perform in this patient?
3. What treatment would you recommend?

This patient almost certainly has an invasive ulcerating squamous cell carcinoma of the cervix uteri. As the lesion appears to be confined to the cervix it would be staged as Ib.

A cervical smear taken in this condition usually reveals frankly malignant cells but a definitive histological diagnosis must still be made on a punch biopsy specimen taken from the edge of the ulcer. Colposcopy will confirm a malignant growth and indicate the best site for a biopsy but is not really necessary when the lesion can be seen with the naked eye.

An examination under anaesthetic should always be performed in cases of invasive carcinoma of the cervix to confirm the preliminary clinical staging so that a decision can be made about the appropriate treatment. Cystoscopy should also be performed to exclude extension to the bladder. An intravenous pyelogram and blood urea estimation will reveal any major ureteric involvement, while a chest X-ray will demonstrate most pulmonary metastases. Lymphangiography to detect pelvic lymph node metastases is rarely used.

Stage Ib carcinoma of the cervix can be treated either with radiotherapy or radical surgery or a combination of both. The former is preferable in older or obese women and was used in this patient. It is, however, contraindicated if there is any evidence of pelvic infection. It usually takes the form of intracavitary treatment with radium or caesium, inserted on two or three occasions, and combined with external irradiation to the pelvic sidewall. The appropriate surgical treatment is a Wertheim's hysterectomy. This involves removal of the uterus, ovaries, fallopian tubes, the parametrial tissue, a cuff of vagina (amounting to at least one third of its length) and a pelvic lymphadenectomy. The operation is usually performed in younger women, or those for whom radiotherapy is either contraindicated or impossible (e.g. vaginal stenosis).

The primary mortality for surgery is higher (approximately 1-3 per cent) and early complications such as ureteric fistulae are more frequent than with radiotherapy. Radiotherapy may, on the other hand, produce late sequelae such as vaginal stenosis, or rectal and bladder ulceration. The five year survival rate following both techniques is similar (approximately 75-80 per cent) and that of combined radiotherapy and surgery a little higher, as is the postoperative morbidity.

27

A 58 year old Irishman who smokes 40 cigarettes a day gives a history of a chronic cough for many years. In winter he brings up purulent sputum which is occasionally bloodstained, and he has episodic fever and ill health. Prior to the present admission, he has lost weight and his breathing has become more difficult.

On examination he has a pyrexia of 39.5°C, is centrally cyanosed and finger clubbing is noted. He is breathless at rest. Chest expansion is poor; the percussion note is impaired in the right axilla and breath sounds, although faint, are vesicular. Crepitations are audible in the right mid zone posteriorly and in the right axilla. Scattered rhonchi are audible.

1. Give four possible causes for haemoptysis in this man.
2. Which of these may be associated with clubbing?

Sputum is sent for 'culture and sensitivity' and the report is 'a mixed growth of organisms'. The chest X-ray shows an opacity in the apical segment of the right lower lobe.

3. Suggest three pathologies accounting for the radiological finding.
4. Give two important investigations.

Haemoptyses in an elderly male who is a heavy smoker warrant immediate investigation for carcinoma of the bronchus or pulmonary tuberculosis. The history in this case is compatible with a diagnosis of chronic bronchitis and frequent infections, which when associated with bronchopneumonia, may lead to haemoptyses. Bronchiectasis developing in an area of previously damaged lung may also give rise to haemoptyses. Finally, patients with chronic lung disease are more prone to venous thromboses and pulmonary emboli — a further cause of haemoptyses, and not always presenting with chest pain.

Chronic pulmonary suppuration, e.g. bronchiectasis and chronic tuberculosis, and bronchial carcinoma are associated with clubbing.

The opacity in the right lower lobe could be due to pneumonic consolidation, pulmonary infarction or a carcinoma.

The most important immediate investigation is to examine sputum for acid fast bacilli and for malignant cells. If neither investigation provides a diagnosis a bronchoscopy should be performed.

28

The patient was a 63 year old solicitor. He complained of a severe pain in the buttocks radiating down both legs associated with unsteadiness on his feet, a sensation of numbness and pins and needles in the feet, and a feeling of general weakness of the legs. These symptoms began suddenly 5 days before admission, and following the acute onset had got rather worse. There was nothing of relevance in his past history except an attack he described as sciatica ten years previously.

On examination he was obese. There were no abnormal physical signs in the cardiovascular system, the respiratory system or the abdomen. Vibration and joint position sensation were absent below mid-calf in both legs, and light touch sensation was impaired over the sole of the right foot and the posterior aspect of the right ankle. Plantar flexion at the right ankle was weaker than on the left. Both ankle jerks were absent. Plantar responses were flexor.

The urine contained no sugar. The chest X-ray and serum B_{12} concentration were both normal. Syphilis serology showed no evidence of treponemal infection. X-rays of the spine showed severe osteoarthritis with osteophyte formation. The L3-4 disc space was greatly narrowed.

1. Where is the lesion in the nervous system?
2. What is the likely cause?
3. What other X-ray examination would you like to see?

The neurological signs in this man point to an affection of motor and sensory functions at or about the level of the S1 dermatome, particularly on the right. Weakness with absent tendon jerks and flexor plantars suggests a lower motor neurone lesion. This could be at any level below the S1 segment of the spinal cord, but, as the lesion is bilateral, it is likely to be above the point where the right and left S1 spinal nerves leave the vertebral canal and become widely separated one from the other. The symptoms of weakness, numbness and paraesthesiae, especially in the feet, would fit with a lesion at this level involving both ventral and dorsal (motor and sensory) roots. Unsteadiness on the feet is likely to be due to impaired joint position sense.

Because the symptoms and signs are both motor and sensory, the lesion is unlikely to be at the spinal cord itself, where motor and sensory roots are separate, but in the cauda equina, where they join together to form the spinal nerve. The pain described by the patient is typical (in both nature and distribution) of an acute compression of the cauda equina.

Compression of the cauda equina is most often due to neoplasm or to a displaced intervertebral disc. The acute onset of symptoms fits best with the latter, and the history of 'sciatica' suggests previous problems with a prolapsed intervertebral disc. Such lesions often occur in osteoarthritic backs, and the X-rays show that the protruding disc is likely to be the one at L3-4, which is in close relation to the S1 spinal nerves.

The next radiological investigation would be myelography: X-rays after introduction of radio-opaque fluid into the subarachnoid space. It was performed in this patient, and showed a prolapsed L3-4 disc causing almost complete occlusion of the vertebral canal. Following the myelogram, the symptoms got worse, and an urgent laminectomy was necessary. Relief of symptoms was complete, and the patient made a full recovery.

29

An 18 year old girl with chronic renal failure had a renal transplant four years ago. Although her overall renal function was good, her blood pressure had remained elevated since the transplant and she required antihypertensive drugs. For the previous six months she had taken bethanidine 20 mg twice daily and hydrochlorthiazide 25 mg once daily which controlled her blood pressure. On the day of admission she had complained of a 'runny nose' and headache. Her local chemist had suggested some tablets which she had taken for the cold. Shortly thereafter she experienced a severe headache, felt nauseous and vomited on several occasions.

On arrival in casualty she was in evident distress with a blood pressure of 190/130 mmHg and pulse rate 100/min, regular. The BP rose to 240/140 mmHg one half hour after admission. The heart was not enlarged and no evidence of cardiac failure was found. Fundoscopy revealed grade II hypertensive changes. Neurological examination was normal.

1. What was the immediate cause of this girl's presentation?
2. Outline briefly the underlying mechanism.
3. How would you lower this girl's blood pressure?

Many proprietary 'cold cures', readily available without prescription at any retail pharmacy, contain symphathomimetic amines. Ephedrine has been largely replaced by its analogue phenylpropanolamine (norephedrine) because of the central stimulant effects of the former. Both these drugs are nasal decongestants.

The cause of the severe hypertensive presentation of this girl is the drug interaction between bethanidine and a sympathomimetic amine. Ephedrine and norephedrine release bethanidine and related drugs from their storage sites within the sympathetic nerve endings and thus reverse the adrenergic neurone blockade allowing the blood pressure to rise. In addition, receptor supersensitivity to sympathomimetic amines occurs in subjects receiving adrenergic blocking drugs and the direct action of ephedrine and related compounds on adrenergic receptors in this situation may be enhanced, thus potentiating the rise in blood pressure.

The presentation constitutes an hypertensive emergency and the blood pressure must be reduced as a matter of urgency. The most logical drug to use in this situation would be an α-blocking agent such as phentolamine, however the duration of action of this drug is very short and other α-blockers such as phenoxybenzamine have an onset of action which is delayed for up to 1-2 hours. The combined α and ß-antagonist, labetolol, administered by intravenous injection would be effective and lowers the arterial pressure within five minutes.

Alternative therapy such as hydralazine (e.g. 25 mg intramuscularly) will lower the blood pressure within 30 minutes. Diazoxide is a more potent vasodilator and great care must be taken to avoid precipitous falls in pressure.

It is advisable to combine a vasodilator with a ß-receptor antagonist to prevent the reflexly mediated sympathetic stimulation, of particular importance in this case.

30

A 15 year old schoolgirl became pregnant as a result of a liaison with an older man and had managed to hide the pregnancy from her parents for six months. She booked at 29 weeks and gave a history of rheumatic mitral incompetence first diagnosed after an episode of congestive cardiac failure three years earlier. At this time she had been treated with digitalis and diuretics. These had subsequently been discontinued although she was still taking prophylactic phenoxymethyl penicillin 125 mg daily. She had remained well since this time with no apparent limitations to her physical activity.

On examination her pulse was regular with a rate of 86 beats per minute, her blood pressure was 130/65 mmHg and her jugular venous pressure was normal. There was no clinical evidence of cardiac enlargement. On auscultation the first heart sound was normal and the second was split. A loud apical pansystolic murmur radiating to the axilla and an ejection murmur in the pulmonary area were heard. The peripheral pulses were normal and no abnormality of the respiratory system was detected.

Abdominal examination revealed that the uterine size and fetus corresponded to a pregnancy of 28 weeks duration. The lie was longitudinal with a cephalic presentation and the fetal heart was audible.

An electrocardiogram was made and this showed a sinus rhythm with 'P' mitrale in Lead I but was otherwise within normal limits.

1. What special precautions would you take during the remaining antenatal period?
2. Describe how you would manage her labour.

During pregnancy this patient should be under the joint care of a cardiac physician and obstetrician and after thirty weeks should be seen weekly in the antenatal clinic. She should also be encouraged to rest as much as possible to minimise the progressive increase in cardiac work which occurs with advancing pregnancy. Routine hospital admission for rest and observation after 36 weeks of pregnancy has been recommended for all pregnant cardiac patients but is not really necessary when there is no significant impairment of physical activities and the patient's social circumstances allow adequate rest at home.

Induction of labour should be avoided in the cardiac patient because of the increased risk associated with intrauterine infection which may occur if labour is prolonged, and also on account of the much higher complication rate associated with Caesarean section in these patients if the attempt at induction fails. In practice most cardiac patients go into spontaneous labour at or near term.

Labour as the word implies involves physical exertion and is a time of increased risk for the woman with cardiac disease. Certain precautions must therefore be observed to minimise the likelihood of cardiac failure. The patient should be encouraged to sit upright with her legs hanging down slightly and the drugs and equipment required to treat acute cardiac failure should be immediately to hand.

To minimise the risk of infection and the grave complications of subacute bacterial endocarditis it is usual to give a broad spectrum prophylactic antibiotic such as cephaloridine or ampicillin during and for five days after labour. Some authorities, however, dispute the need for this while others recommend more powerful combinations such as penicillin and streptomycin or ampicillin and gentamicin.

Pain is stressful and imposes an added strain on the patient. Adequate analgesia is therefore essential. An epidural should be used if necessary but it is vital to avoid hypotension, as the diseased heart is unable to compensate for this by increasing its output.

If oxytocin is necessary this should be given using an infusion pump to avoid administering large volumes of fluid. This drug has an antidiuretic action and it is therefore important to monitor fluid balance carefully.

The second stage of labour should be kept as short as possible and forceps delivery should be performed as a routine to minimise the effort required by the patient.

Ergometrine must not be given as a rapid rise in central venous pressure follows its use and predisposes to cardiac failure. Many obstetricians prefer to avoid oxytocics altogether in their management of the third stage but an intramuscular injection or intravenous bolus of 5 units of oxytocin is acceptable.

31

The patient was aged 42, childless, separated from her husband. She worked as a receptionist for a fashionable private doctor, who sent her to see one of his colleagues at her request because of excessive hair growth on her arms. This had been present for many years, but she had only recently worried about it. She had been in hospital twice. The first time was soon after marriage at the age of 26, with a psychiatric illness that she refused to discuss: the second admission, aged 37, was for investigation for a malignant growth, which the doctors had suspected might be present but were unable to find. She said she was fit apart from the excess body hair, ate well, drank no alcohol, and took regular exercise. On direct questioning she revealed that she had had amenorrhoea for five years in her twenties, again at the time of her second hospital admission, and also for the last seven months. She denied any symptoms related to the gut, but said she was worried in case she had renal failure.

On examination she was of normal height (1.65 m) but was very light (29 kg). She was grossly wasted, with loss of muscle bulk and no subcutaneous fat on the body, although the breasts were well preserved. The hair of which she complained was visible on her arms and back and was fine, soft, short and white. The head, pubic and axillary hair were normal. There were no other abnormal signs. Because she was worried about renal failure, the practice nurse had sent plasma for electrolytes and urea: the results were — sodium 134 mmol/l, potassium 2.7 mmol/l and urea 1.4 mmol/l (normal 2.5-6.6 mmol/l).

1. What is the most likely diagnosis and why?
2. Suggest four other diagnoses that must be excluded.
3. Comment on the blood results.

The physical signs in this patient are those of starvation. The fine, downy, 'lanugo' hair of which she complains is a feature (mechanism unknown) of starvation itself, not of any underlying wasting illness. There are many points that lead to the diagnosis of anorexia nervosa, which has probably been intermittently present since at least the age of 26. These include the history of psychiatric illness of uncertain nature, particularly as that occurred around the time of her marriage: social or sexual stress sometimes precipitate the disease. The illness at 37 sound as though she was wasted, and that a sinister non-psychiatric cause was wrongly suspected. Amenorrhoea has occurred with each relapse, and this is usual in anorexia nervosa. Claiming to be fit, and taking regular exercise although starved are said to be typical of this condition, and the rationalisation of her problem as 'renal failure' suggests that she is either deluded or manipulative. A final point is that in anorexia nervosa, breast tissue, and pubic and axillary hair, are well preserved, unlike wasting illnesses of known organic cause.

Alternative diagnoses are such wasting illnesses. It would be negligent (as in any physical examination) to omit to test the urine for sugar, in case the weight loss is due to diabetes mellitus. Other endocrine disorders sometimes confused with anorexia nervosa are hypopituitarism — where pubic and axillary hair are lost and breasts are atrophic — and Addison's disease, which might produce pigmentation and would give a different electrolyte picture. Diseases of the gut with wasting include malabsorption of any kind, and particularly Crohn's disease. An occult carcinoma is a diagnosis which has already been considered, and lymphoma is also a possibility. The difficult and important decision is the extent to which an organic disease should be sought by investigation: unnecessarily prolonged and complicated investigations may reinforce the idea of an 'organic' disease in the patient's delusional structure, and make psychiatric treatment more difficult.

The electrolyte and urea changes are due to starvation. Circulating urea is largely derived from protein in the diet, and a urea of 1.4 mmol/l is diagnostic of a diet with very little or no protein. There is also a trend to mild hyponatraemia and mild hypokalaemia with starvation.

32

A 54 year old night club owner was brought into the casualty department at 4 a.m. with a complaint of severe abdominal pain. He admitted to having experienced a similar but less severe pain intermittently for the past year. Latterly it had occurred approximately three days per week, was intermittent in nature and situated in the upper half of the abdomen and radiating occasionally through to the back.

On this occasion the pain had been present for two days increasing in severity and associated with nausea and vomiting. In addition he admitted to variable diarrhoea for the past six months. His bowels were open seven or eight times per day but the stools contained neither blood nor mucous.

He smoked 60 cigarettes per day and drank alcohol in excess.

On examination he was observed to be an obese individual in great pain and sweating profusely. He was neither anaemic nor icteric. Gynaecomastia was present and he had palmar erythema. The pulse was 96/min and regular, BP 110/75 mmHg, JVP not elevated and the heart was clinically normal. There were no abnormal signs in the lung fields. In the abdomen the liver was palpable 5 cm below the costal margin and the spleen tip was felt. There was marked tenderness with guarding most evident in the epigastrium. Bowel sounds were absent, rectal examination was normal and stools were negative for occult blood.

1. Give three causes for the abdominal pain.
2. What other conditions may be present and what is the evidence?
3. List the three most urgent investigations.
4. Outline your initial treatment of this case assuming your most probable diagnosis is correct.

The physical signs elicited on examination of this man indicate the development of peritonitis. The long history of pain in a person who imbibes excessive quantities of alcohol makes the diagnosis of pancreatitis probable. However, alcoholics are more susceptible than non-drinkers to peptic ulceration, and the history of recurrent pain radiating through to the back could indicate a posterior duodenal ulcer which in this case may well have perforated.

Other causes of a similar presentation should be considered such as acute cholecystitis with rupture of the gall bladder. A leaking abdominal aneurysm may present in this way.

The history of alcohol abuse and the findings of hepatomegaly, splenomegaly, palmar erythema and gynaecomastia indicate chronic liver disease (alcoholic cirrhosis).

Persistent diarrhoea in the absence of signs of gastrointestinal blood loss in this patient could well be due to chronic pancreatic disease, in which case biochemical evidence of malabsorption may be found on investigation.

Urgent investigations are aimed at establishing the diagnosis and determining the overall state of hydration of the patient. Thus a serum amylase, erect and supine X-ray of the abdomen, full blood count and blood urea and electrolytes should be performed. (In this case the amylase was grossly raised and the abdominal films revealed pancreatic calcification).

Conservative management of pancreatitis in the first instance is advocated and treatment is aimed at restoring adequate fluid balance with intravenous fluids and controlling pain with analgesics. A nasogastric tube should be inserted with aspiration of gastric juices.

For severe pain pethidine or morphine may be required but both cause spasm of the sphincter of Oddi (morphine more than pethidine). Hypocalcaemia may complicate pancreatitis and intravenous calcium gluconate is required in such cases.

If the initial investigations indicate a perforated ulcer, i.v. fluids and nasogastric suction are established, blood is crossmatched and a laparotomy must be performed.

33

A 30 year old Indian woman, who became pregnant for the first time after artificial insemination by a donor, booked for antenatal care at 18 weeks of pregnancy. At this time she complained of morning sickness and was treated with an antiemetic. She also complained of an irritant vaginal discharge which had not improved after treatment with cream which she had obtained from her GP. A monilial vaginitis was diagnosed and nystatin pessaries prescribed. Her discharge and morning sickness thereafter improved rapidly. The pregnancy subsequently progressed normally until 30 weeks when she was admitted to hospital because of a brown vaginal discharge which had been present for two days and a painless vaginal blood loss (about half a cup full) which had occurred on the morning of admission.

On examination she appeared fit and was not shocked or anaemic. Her pulse rate was 80 beats per minute and blood pressure 140/95 mmHg. Her uterus was enlarged to 30 weeks size. The fetal lie was clearly longitudinal with a high free cephalic presentation. The fetal heart was heard easily and was of normal rate and rhythm. There was no oedema and urine analysis was normal. Her haemoglobin was 11.0 g/dl.

1. What further examination and investigations would you perform?
2. What are the possible causes of her bleeding?
3. What is the treatment of the most likely causes?

This patient has experienced an antepartum haemorrhage and a vaginal examination is therefore contraindicated. A speculum examination is permissible, however, and should be performed when the bleeding has subsided in order to exclude a local cause such as a cervical polyp, an erosion or (very rarely) malignancy.

It is important to differentiate between the inevitable bleeding of a placenta praevia and a revealed accidental haemorrhage or *abruptio placentae*. In this patient the absence of pain, the lack of uterine tenderness and easily felt fetus all suggest a possible placenta praevia. The high presenting part is also suspicious but is not uncommon at this stage in a normal pregnancy.

The best method for diagnosing a placenta praevia is ultrasound scanning. In skilled hands this can be used to locate the placenta with some accuracy. Older methods such as isotopic scanning, and radiographic techniques are less satisfactory and are rarely used nowadays. This patient was found to have a complete or Type III placenta praevia when ultrasound scanning was performed. All patients with a placenta praevia must be kept in hospital as bleeding may be recurrent and can be severe. Blood should be cross matched and available for transfusion when necessary. Provided heavy bleeding does not occur the pregnancy should be allowed to continue to 38 weeks. Traditionally an examination under anaesthetic should be performed at this time with full preparation for a Caesarean section if a major degree (Type II, III or IV) of placenta praevia is confirmed. Reliable ultrasound evidence of the placental site makes this procedure both unnecessary and potentially hazardous and an elective Caesarean section without EUA is preferable. If the placenta praevia is lateral (Type I) then EUA and artificial rupture of the membranes is advisable.

Fetal pulmonary maturity should be confirmed beforehand by amniotic fluid lecithin/sphingomyelin ratio estimation if there is doubt about the gestational age of the fetus. (The amniocentesis should be done under ultrasound control).

In the event that a minor placental abruption is diagnosed, continuous fetal heart monitoring (for example, by phonocardiography or ultrasound) should be carried out to exclude fetal distress produced by placental separation. Fetal distress is an indication for immediate Caesarean section, but otherwise the management can be conservative and the onset of spontaneous labour awaited, bearing in mind the greater likelihood of further abruption and/or fetal distress in labour.

34

A 60 year old lady had consulted her doctor intermittently for the past three years with painful joints. Initially she had complained of pain in the knees, shoulders and wrists, more marked on awakening in the morning. The general practitioner had prescribed mild analgesics with some benefit. For several months she would be free from pain, but the joint symptoms would return and latterly had affected her fingers and both temperomandibular joints.

Three weeks prior to admission she developed a fever, felt unwell and experienced a sharp pain in the left axillary region, which was exacerbated by breathing. She denied a cough or the production of sputum. These symptoms were present until the time of admission and had not been relieved by a course of a broad spectrum antibiotic.

On examination she was febrile with a macular rash confined to both cheeks and extending over the bridge of the nose. Respiration was shallow and restricted by pain in the left chest.

There were no abnormalities in the cardiovascular, alimentary or central nervous systems. In the chest, air entry was reduced at the left base where crepitations were audible, and a pleural rub was heard in the left axilla.

Metacarpophalangeal, wrist, shoulder, knee and temperomandibular joints were painful with passive movement. However, there was no demonstrable swelling, increase in temperature or deformity.

1. Suggest possible causes for her joint pains?
2. How do you account for the pleuritic pain?
3. What investigations are indicated?

There are multiple causes for joint pains in the elderly and osteoarthritis is common in this age group. However, the history in this case suggests alternative possibilities. The remission and relapse of symptoms and the distribution of the joints affected make a diagnosis of osteoarthritis less probable.

Rheumatoid arthritis and related conditions often present with intermittent joint involvement, and frequently pain most evident in the morning on rising. Characteristic involvement of the hand by rheumatoid may progress to a classical deformity which includes metacarpophalangeal swelling and deformity, subluxation of joints, and ulnar deviation at the wrist.

The long history militates against infective causes. Gout must however, be considered.

Pleuritic pain may have occurred as a response to infection, underlying infarction of the lung due to embolism or involvement by a malignant process. There are few clues as to which of these is most likely, nevertheless, it is always appropriate to account for all presenting symptoms and signs with a single diagnosis. Thus a history of joint involvement of a 'rheumatoid type', a pleuritic illness and a rash with a butterfly distribution on the face raises the possibility of systemic lupus erythematosus.

Investigations should be directed towards the nature of the joint involvement, the cause of the chest pain and the underlying illness. Thus X-rays of the involved joints, serum uric acid and tests for rheumatoid arthritis and systemic lupus (R.A. Latex, rheumatoid factor, L.E. cells, antinuclear factor, etc) should be performed. A chest X-ray, sputum culture and where indicated a lung scan must be arranged.

Multisystem involvement is common with systemic lupus and the kidneys may be affected (proteinuria). Anti-DNA antibodies can be identified in the serum of most patients.

35

You are telephoned by the casualty officer, who says he has seen a man with a myocardial infarct, and has given him diamorphine because the pain is so severe.

When the patient arrives in the Coronary Care Unit you elicit the following history. He is a 48 year old self-employed long distance lorry driver, and is about 200 miles away from his home. The pain, which began while he was dining in a restaurant, is severe, crushing in quality, and radiates from the centre of the chest to the jaw and left arm. The only event of note in the past history is a road traffic accident, in which he was saved from asphyxia by an emergency tracheostomy performed by a policeman. He says he was in hospital for some time following that accident, and was discharged 6 months ago.

On examination, the only abnormal signs are a scar over the trachea, and a number of scars of intravenous infusions — these are apparently because he was fed intravenously for some weeks after the road traffic accident. He is in sinus rhythm, and is not in cardiac failure. The e.c.g. shows no abnormality.

During the night the pain is controlled by a further three injections of diamorphine, but apart from pain he is very well, and there is no arrhythmia. However, when the sister comes on duty the next morning she finds him smoking a cigarette while wearing his oxygen mask. When she warns him of the danger, he replies with a torrent of abuse, tears the electrodes off his chest, dresses and strides out of the hospital.

1. What do you suspect?
2. Was the casualty officer right to give diamorphine?

There is nothing in this case history to prove that the diagnosis of myocardial infarction was wrong. The pain is typical, and a normal e.c.g. on admission does not rule out the diagnosis. However, it is very unusual for patients with a recent myocardial infarction to feel well and energetic enough to take their own discharge.

In retrospect, there are a number of other unusual features. One should always be a little suspicious of patients who are said to be a long way away from home when they seek help: this is sometimes a device used by patients to cover their tracks. The history of the road traffic accident certainly corresponds to the signs, but why should asphyxia that was relieved by tracheostomy need prolonged and many-sited intravenous infusions? The complete absence of physical and electrocardiographic signs of myocardial infarction is certainly odd. Finally, analgesia with diamorphine seems to be particularly important for this patient.

These all suggest that our patient may have simulated his story to obtain narcotics, and that he left at about the time when suspicions would start to be voiced. He may have developed a taste for opiates when his throat was injured, but even the history of injury may be a fabrication, and the tracheostomy may have been done for another reason — for example, for prolonged ventilation after a narcotic overdose. The numerous intravenous injection sites might suggest that he has frequently been successful in getting the treatment he wants.

However, the casualty officer did not have the benefit of the complete story, and was probably right to prescribe diamorphine. It is arguably a more venial fault to omit to give adequate analgesia to a patient in pain than it is to be taken in by a drug abuser, who, if he is not successful with you, will succeed elsewhere. If one cannot believe the patient then who can be believed?

36

Two patients were admitted complaining of difficulty in swallowing.

The first was an 82 year old woman. She had presented to the outpatients department one year previously complaining of upper abdominal pain and heartburn. Barium studies at that time had shown an hiatus hernia. For two or three months before admission she had noticed that food seemed to stick at the lower end of the sternum, and for 6 weeks she had regurgitated food 2 or 3 minutes after each mouthful. The problem was getting steadily worse but there had been no difficulty in swallowing fluids.

The second patient was a 67 year old jeweller. His symptoms had begun suddenly. When he tried to swallow he spluttered and choked. If he tried to swallow fluids, some of the fluid would come back through his nose. His voice had become faint and hoarse. On examination, the palate moved to the right, rather than elevating centrally, and when he tried to put out his tongue, it deviated to the left. Indirect laryngoscopy showed that the left vocal cord was paralysed.

1. Give at least two possible diagnoses in the first case. Which investigations would be most helpful?
2. Where is the lesion in the second case?

Difficulties with swallowing may be due to abnormalities of structure in the upper gut, or abnormalities of its function. These cases illustrate both problems.

The history of a sensation of food sticking or catching on the way down is characteristic of a structural lesion, and the gradual increase in severity of the symptom suggests a progressive pathology. The localisation of the symptom to the level of the lower end of the sternum may point to an obstruction at the lower end of the oesophagus. A past history of hiatus hernia would fit with a peptic stricture of the oesophagus, but carcinoma of the oesophagus could present with exactly the same symptoms, including regurgitation of food recently swallowed. Vomiting of food eaten hours or days previously might be due to an obstruction further on in the gastrointestinal tract, such as the pyloric end of the stomach. Achalasia of the cardia is a third possibility in the first patient, but is less likely to present at this age than a malignant or fibrotic stricture.

A structural lesion must be seen, either directly or on X-ray, for the diagnosis to be made. The first investigation in such a case as this would usually be a barium swallow, and this would be followed by fibreoptic oesophagoscopy under local anaesthetic.

In the second case a neurological abnormality has caused disorder in the functions of the pharyngeal muscles involved in swallowing, and there is a laryngeal palsy with dysphonia. The problem with fluids returning through the nose is because of failure of the palate to close off the nasopharynx from the oropharynx as intrapharyngeal pressure rises during the act of swallowing, and a similar failure to close off the larynx has led to spluttering and choking. The physical examination has shown palsies of the ninth, tenth and twelfth cranial nerves, and if a single lesion is to be proposed it must be where these nerves or their nuclei are close together: possible sites include the left anterior portion of the medulla oblongata (for the nuclei) or just beneath the base of the skull as the nerves emerge.

In the first case, barium swallow examination showed a carcinoma of the oesophagus, and biopsy through the fibreoptic oesophagoscope showed that the tumour was highly undifferentiated. The acute onset of symptoms in the second case suggested a vascular lesion, but the problem was, surprisingly, infiltration of the meninges around the medulla with secondary carcinoma from a primary in the prostate gland.

37

A 21 year old female medical student returned from a party in the early hours of the morning. She slept well for several hours but woke with a nagging pain in her abdomen. She attributed the pain to the previous evening's indiscretion, however, over the next few hours the pain increased in intensity and she felt generally unwell with nausea and vomited on two occasions a small quantity of unremarkable fluid. There was no diarrhoea. The pain was persistent in character with exacerbations of increased severity and described as 'central abdominal pain'. She had a normal bowel motion the previous day.

In the afternoon she presented herself to the casualty officer who elicited the following signs on examination.

Pyrexia 38.5°C, pulse 90/min; BP 120/70 mmHg; heart and lungs normal. The tongue was furred and, on examination of the abdomen, there was no distension but tenderness with guarding was elicited to the right of the umbilicus. No masses were palpable and bowel sounds were normal. Rectal examination revealed no abnormality.

Investigations showed: Hb 13 g/dl and WBC 13 x 10^9/l. X-ray of the abdomen was normal.

1. Give a differential diagnosis for the abdominal pain.
2. What further history is important to elicit?
3. What additional investigations are required?
4. How would you treat this girl's illness?

This girl presents with an acute abdomen which is unlikely to be related to the previous evening's 'indiscretion'.

The mild pyrexia and abdominal signs indicate an underlying inflammatory process with localised peritonitism for which there may be several causes. However, acute appendicitis must be considered a likely diagnosis. Unlike the textbook descriptions of an acute appendix, many cases present with far from classical signs, in part due to the variable position of the appendix (e.g. retrocaecal, pelvic, postileal).

In many cases, tenderness is elicited on rectal examination but this was not observed in this case.

Other conditions with a similar presentation include acute cholecystitis, Crohn's disease, infection of the genitourinary system, e.g. salpingitis, pyelonephritis, ureteric colic and complications of early pregnancy e.g. ectopic pregnancy.

It is imperative that an accurate menstrual history be obtained in addition a history of any relevant urinary systems. The urine should be examined in all cases. Light microscopy of an uncentrifuged urine may reveal inflammatory cells which provides a diagnosis long before the results of culture become available.

If the diagnosis of acute appendix is considered most likely, a laparotomy should be performed without delay. In the event of uncertainty and in the presence of localised signs and negative urinary microscopy, a laparotomy must still be carried out.

38

A 51 year old nulliparous computer clerk attended the gynaecology outpatient clinic complaining of heavy, prolonged, irregular and infrequent periods for six months. Before this menstruation had been regular with four days bleeding every 28 days. Her first abnormal period had lasted 14 days. It had been followed by three months amenorrhoea and then a second very heavy bleed lasting for four days. She then had two normal periods and a month later again experienced a heavy 14 day vaginal bleed with the passage of clots. There had not been any dysmenorrhoea nor any intermenstrual bleeding. She had never had sexual intercourse and there was no history of hot flushes or hormone therapy. She was otherwise well but gave a history of pulmonary tuberculosis 32 years earlier. She also suffered from epilepsy and was taking phenytoin and phenobarbitone.

On examination she was rather obese and moderately hypertensive with a blood pressure of 160/100 mmHg. There was no abnormality of her breasts or adbomen. Inspection of her vulva and vagina revealed profuse watery, yellow-brown vaginal discharge but no sign of vaginitis. Her cervix was nulliparous and healthy. On bimanual examination the uterus felt bulky and irregular but was anteverted and mobile. Neither ovary was palpable and there were no adnexal masses. Investigations: cervical smear — no evidence of malignancy. Many leucocytes and groups of active columnar cells which were endometrial in type were present. High vaginal swab culture — no bacterial pathogen, monilia or Trichomonas vaginalis was identified. Haemoglobin — 10.2 g/dl.

1. Describe the normal menopause.
2. Give a differential diagnosis for this patient's perimenopausal irregular vaginal bleeding.
3. What investigation would you perform to establish the cause?

Although menstruation may simply stop abruptly, the normal menopause usually involves either a gradual diminution in menstrual flow with regular cycles or an increasing number of 'missed' periods until eventually they cease altogether. The average age of the menopause is 50 years but it may occur as early as 40 or as late as 55 years.

The irregular, prolonged and heavy bleeding experienced by this patient is therefore abnormal. The most likely cause is 'metropathia haemorrhagica' a form of dysfunctional bleeding (i.e. without an organic disease of the genital tract) which is common at the two extremes of the reproductive period of a woman's life. It is due to unopposed oestrogen stimulation of the endometrium associated with anovulatory cycles. Clinically it usually produces two to three months amenorrhoea followed by prolonged painless heavy bleeding. Histological examination reveals that this is due to the breakdown of a thickened endometrium showing cystic hyperplasia. When the cysts are large the naked eye appearance of the endometrium may resemble 'Swiss gruyere cheese'. Bleeding in this condition may be so prolonged and heavy that it is life threatening.

The irregular uterus of this patient suggested the possibility of fibroids. When they are submucus these tumours can certainly cause menorrhagia but do not usually disrupt the menstrual cycle. Adenomyosis may also cause an enlarged, irregular uterus and menorrhagia but the bleeding is usually associated with congestive dysmenorrhoea which was absent in the case described. Benign endometrial polyps and fibroid polyps can cause menorrhagia and intermenstrual bleeding but the latter are usually associated with abdominal pain. Endometrial adenocarcinoma (carcinoma of the corpus uteri) clasically causes postmenopausal bleeding but may also cause menorrhagia and intermenstrual bleeding. This malignant tumour and the very much less common sarcoma of the uterus must always be borne in mind in cases of irregular perimenopausal bleeding, because although not as common as the causes enumerated above, they are clearly of far more sinister significance.

A careful examination under anaesthetic and diagnostic curettage *must always* be performed to exclude malignant disease. This patient has many of the features characteristic of the women at risk of developing endometrial adenocarcinoma *viz* nulliparity, hypertension and age greater than 50 years. Indeed histology revealed that she had a well differentiated endometrial adenocarcinoma and her treatment consisted of an extended abdominal hysterectory. This involved removal of both ovaries, fallopian tubes, the uterus, and after dissection of the ureters 3 cm cuff of vagina. The tumour was found to have spread directly to within 2 mm of the pelvic peritoneum and post operative external irradiation was therefore given.

39

A 20 year old office clerk consulted his G.P., when for two days he had experienced painful aching wrist and knee joints. The doctor prescribed indomethacin tablets which partially relieved the symptoms, but for a period of six days the wrists, elbows, knees, shoulders and temperomandibular joints were symmetrically involved with pain and stiffness, especially in the early morning. The joint symptoms resolved, but ten days later he again consulted his doctor and, on this occasion, was frankly jaundiced. He admitted to passing dark coloured urine and his stools were pale. He was anorectic and generally unwell. Physical examination confirmed the icterus and revealed a slightly enlarged tender liver. There were no signs of chronic liver disease.

Preliminary investigations showed: Hb — 14 g/dl; WBC — 6.0 x 10^9/l; bilirubin — 80μmol/l (5-17); aspartate aminotransferase — 95 iu (5-30); alkaline phosphatase — 60 iu (20-95); chest X-ray — normal; urinalysis — bilirubin present in excess.

1. Give three possible diagnoses for the joint symptoms, which the G.P. might have considered at the first consultation.
2. Suggest three causes for the subsequent development of jaundice.
3. What single further investigation would you request?
4. If jaundice continued and protein electrophoresis revealed albumin 40 g/l, globulin 70 g/l, suggest a further possible diagnosis and two appropriate investigations.

An acute symmetrical polyarthralgia or arthritis developing in a young person has several possible causes. Rheumatoid arthritis may present in this way and characteristically the joints are stiff and more painful in the early morning. Symmetrical involvement of the joints is not a feature of acute rheumatic fever. Polyarthralgia may occur in the prodromal period of several infectious illnesses, such as rubella, infectious monomucleosis and hepatitis. It also occurs with brucellosis, typhoid fever and Reiters syndrome.

The development of jaundice in a young person is most likely to be due to an infective agent. In the U.K., infective hepatitis or serum jaundice are the commonest agents. The clinical observations and investigations suggest a hepatocellular jaundice with obstructive features. The latter is frequently associated with viral hepatitis, but other causes such as drug induced jaundice (e.g. phenothiazines) should be considered. Other hepatotoxins particularly paracetamol when taken in excessive dosage are now well recognised. The predromal symptoms and the age of the patient make other causes of obstructive jaundice less likely (e.g. biliary obstruction secondary to gallstones).

The most important investigation at this stage would be investigation of serum for Australia antigen.

If the condition progresses and protein electrophoresis reveals a grossly elevated globulin fraction, a possible diagnosis of chronic active hepatitis should be made, in which case differential immunoglobulin studies would reveal a grossly elevated IgG and mitochondrial antibodies would be found at high titre in the serum.

40

The daughter of a pit deputy in Yorkshire commenced regular sexual intercourse at the age of 14 years, the year in which her periods started. She left school at the age of 15 years and trained as a secretary. She never used any contraception and became pregnant at the age of 20 years. She presented to her family practitioner at 22 weeks gestation, and her request for a termination of the pregnancy was refused. At 30 weeks gestation, she moved to London to avoid local scandal. She stayed in a 'bed-sitter' and ate predominantly beans on toast and food 'from a take-away'. She booked at 32 weeks. On examination, the pregnancy appeared to be normal, but the routine blood tests showed the following:

Hb 9.4 g/dl, PCV 0.279, MCV 85 fl, MCH 28 pg, MCHC 33.8 g, Hb/dl.

1. What further investigations would you perform?
2. What was the probable cause of her anaemia?
3. How would you treat it?

The correct initial investigations of this normocytic, normochromic anaemia are a serum iron and a total iron binding capacity measurement. The results were 10 μmol/1 (low) and 89 μmol/1 (high) respectively. These results confirmed the probable diagnosis of an iron deficiency anaemia. In its more severe degrees this type of anaemia will produce a microcytic hypochromic picture, but in pregnancy it is common to find a mild form in which the MCV and the MCH are just within the limits of the normal range. If the serum iron and the T.I.B.C. had been equivocal, the next step would have been a bone marrow puncture to examine erythropoietic precursors and marrow iron stores.

Less commonly in pregnancy, anaemia may present a macrocytic picture. This is almost invariably due to a folate deficiency. Treatment with folic acid 10-15 mg daily should be curative. Vitamin B_{12} deficiency is very rare in pregnancy and the possibility can be ignored unless the patient has gastrointestinal symptoms. (Note — in patients with a Mediterranean or negroid ancestry, anaemia may be due to haemoglobin abnormalities and routine haemoglobin electrophoresis should be performed).

The best treatment of iron deficiency anaemia is with oral iron such as ferrous fumarate 200 mg three times a day (ferrous sulphate is cheaper, but tends to cause nausea in pregnancy — ferrous gluconate is a satisfactory alternative). If as in this case, the patient cannot be relied upon to take the tablets, iron injections (Jectofer — iron sorbitol/citric acid complex) can be given. This is preferable to 'total dose infusions' of intravenous iron dextran (Imferon) since the haemopoietic response is equally rapid and it avoids the risk of anaphylactic reactions which is present with the intravenous route.

41

A 49 year old commercial artist had suffered from rheumatoid arthritis for four years. His joints had been painful for most of that time despite treatment with aspirin, two courses of gold injections, phenylbutazone and indomethacin: at times he had been unable to hold a pencil. He had lost 8 kg in weight over the last six months.

He presented to the rheumatologist with a three day history of mild central chest pain unrelated to food, respiration or exercise. He was admitted to hospital and clerked by a medical student. The only abnormal physical signs apart from joint swelling and deformity were dullness to percussion at the right base rising into the right axilla and absent breath sounds in the same area.

The next day a consultant physician found the same signs and also a noise audible over the praecordium, starting early in systole and extending to the middle of diastole, heard best with the patient sitting forward.

1. What is the diagnosis?
2. Do you think the student was remiss not to have found the same signs as the consultant?
3. Suggest at least six useful investigations.

The physical signs in the chest are those of a pleural effusion, which may be due to rheumatoid arthritis or to a second illness such as infection or neoplasm. The chest pain is not pleuritic in type, and is therefore unlikely to be related to the pleural effusion: however, the noise over the praeocrdium is typical of the friction rub of pericarditis, which can produce a pain such as the patient describes. Pericarditis can be due to the inflammation of serous membranes found in rheumatoid disease, but other causes such as virus infection or myocardial infarction must not be ignored. The weight loss may be due only to the rheumatoid disease but should alert you to the possibility of neoplasm or chronic infection (such as tuberculosis) as a cause of the effusion.

Pericardial friction rubs are notably evanescent, and the noise may indeed have been absent when the student made his physical examination. However, he should have been alerted by the unexplained symptom and repeated examination of the heart would have been worthwhile.

An e.c.g. is needed to look for both the widespread, concave-upwards S-T segment elevation and T-wave inversion of pericarditis, and for any cardiographic evidence of recent myocardial infarction. If there was a 'silent' myocardial infarct at around the time that the pain began the cardiac enzymes, especially the lactate dehydrogenase and the hydroxybutyric dehydrogenase, might still be elevated, and these should be estimated. A chest X-ray, both posteroanterior and right lateral, will confirm the presence of the effusion and might show any underlying neoplasm or infection. The most direct method to find the aetiology of the effusion is aspiration of the pleural fluid, followed by examination for rheumatoid factor, and malignant cells, and culture including culture for tubercle bacilli. A Mantoux test should be performed. Other blood investigations are of less diagnostic importance, but a blood count may show the anaemia often found in longstanding rheumatoid disease, and any leucocytosis should be noted. The ESR will inevitably be elevated in a patient with active rheumatoid arthritis, but the estimation is still worthwhile as an assessment of the activity of the disease. Viral antibody titres against viruses likely to cause pericarditis, such as Coxsackie viruses, should be measured.

42

A 30 year old man is admitted to hospital with a history of continuous wheezing and breathlessness for four days. He had had frequent attacks of asthma since childhood and had recently been prescribed bronchodilator drugs by his general practitioner. On examination he was in considerable distress with great difficulty breathing.

1. What five clinical signs would be important in assessing the severity of this patient's asthma?
2. Two important and immediate investigations are indicated. What are these?
3. Outline your immediate management of this patient?

This man gives a long history of asthma since childhood, which suggests that his disease is of the 'atopic' type and a strong family history of allergic conditions is likely.

The frequency of his attacks and his current prolonged breathlessness should alert the admitting physician. Status asthmaticus constitutes a medical emergency and fatalities occur not uncommonly. The five important clinical signs which indicate the severity of the condition are cyanosis which indicates anoxia; a tachycardia reflecting cardiac embarrassment due either to the anoxia or to the injudicious use of sympathomimetic bronchodilator drugs; pulsus paradoxus; dehydration, resulting from hyperventilation and reduced fluid intake, and exhaustion.

Of all possible investigations, arterial blood gas analysis is the most vital. Cyanosis is a difficult physical sign to elicit particularly in the 'coloured' patient and the determination of the arterial Po_2 and Pco_2 is mandatory. Early in the asthmatic attack the Pco_2 is normal or low but a raised Pco_2 is an indication of severe respiratory distress.

A pneumothorax may complicate severe asthma, and require specific management, thus a chest X-ray must be performed.

With severe asthma, not responsive to bronchodilator drugs, immediate therapy must be instigated. Humidified oxygen should be administered by mask in the presence of anoxia. If the pCO_2 is raised a trial of 24 per cent O_2 by ventimask is reasonable (but should improvement in the condition not occur, intermittent positive pressure respiration (IPPR) must be initiated). A tachycardia greater than 130/min is a contraindication to the use of sympathomimetic drugs, however, if the pulse rate is less than this value, i.v. aminophylline or salbutamol should be administered by slow injection. In status asthmaticus steroids should be administered as soon as the diagnosis is established. Rehydration with intravenous fluids may be indicated, and when exhaustion of the patient supervenes, IPPR must be initiated without delay.

43

The patient's husband telephoned her doctor at midnight on Christmas Eve. The history was as follows: his wife had had no trouble with her eyes, and only wore glasses for reading, until a few weeks earlier, when she noticed that street lights appeared fuzzy, 'like the moon seen through a haze'. They had spent the earlier part of the evening celebrating the Season with a few drinks in their local, but soon after they set out for home at 8 o'clock she felt severe pain in and around her right eye. When they got home her husband tried to look at the affected eye, but could hardly do so, because it was uncomfortable to have a torch shone in the eye. As far as the doctor could tell from the telephone description, the eye was red, the cornea cloudy and the pupil dilated. The pain was no better, and the patient was desperate for help.

The doctor had hardly ever met the patient, because she was very healthy for her 71 years, but he made the correct diagnosis from the above history.

1. What is the correct diagnosis, and why did the attack occur in the evening?
2. What initial treatment should be prescribed?
3. What are the other two common causes of a painful red eye?

This story is typical of acute 'closed angle' glaucoma. The patient must have eyes with a narrow anterior chamber, and the iris must have obstructed the outflow of aqueous humour from the anterior chamber into the canal of Schlemm, causing a rise in intraocular pressure. The prodromal attacks, seeing haloes around lights, are typical and are due to temporary rises in intraocular pressure with oedema of the cornea. Attacks typically occur in the evening: in this case, stepping out of the local public house into the dark probably caused pupillary dilatation: the iris is thicker when the pupil dilates, and is therefore more likely to obstruct the flow of aqueous. In the full attack described, the obstruction is complete, so the intraocular pressure rises steeply, with severe pain and vascular congestion. The pupil is stuck down in its dilated position, and there is corneal oedema, as seen by the patient's husband: if he had been allowed to touch the eye he would have detected that it was rock hard.

There are three points to note in the acute treatment. The first is that the pain is severe, and analgesics must be prescribed. The second is that miotic eye drops should be instilled, to constrict the pupil and thus to lift the obstructing iris from the angle of the anterior chamber. Third, acetazolamide can be given to inhibit formation of aqueous humour.

The other leading causes of a painful red eye are acute conjunctivitis and acute iritis: they can both occur in the young, unlike acute glaucoma. Acute conjunctivitis may be bilateral, and behind the infected conjunctivae the internal structures of the eye are normal. Acute iritis gives marked photophobia, inflammatory changes visible within the eye, and typically a constricted pupil.

44

A woman of 64 years had been in remarkably good health all her life. Some months previously she had had a two day illness associated with diarrhoea. For the past six weeks she had found it increasingly difficult to open her bowels and often several days would elapse between bowel motions. The stools were a normal colour.

At the time of referral to the clinic she had last defaecated six days previously. She complained of increasing left sided abdominal pain, intermittent in nature and felt nauseous and had vomited several times in the last three days. In addition, she had lost 8 kg in weight during the past two months.

On examination, she was much distressed by the pain. She was not clinically anaemic and there was no lymphadenopathy. The heart and lungs were clinically normal, and there were no abnormalities on examination of the central nervous system.

The abdomen was distended and tense, but no dullness was elicited in the flanks. Neither liver, kidneys nor spleen were palpable, but the descending colon was palpable and considered to be loaded with faeces. Bowel sounds were increased in intensity. Rectal examination revealed no abnormality.

1. Outline the immediate investigations you would carry out.
2. How would the results of these investigations influence your management of this case?
3. What is the most likely diagnosis and give two alternative diagnoses.

This patient presents with intestinal obstruction (constipation, vomiting and abdominal pain with distension). The order of priorities for investigation are to determine the extent of fluid and electrolyte loss (since she has been vomiting for several days), localise the site of the obstruction, and determine its cause.

Thus initially a blood urea and serum electrolytes should be done together with a haemoglobin and PCV, to determine the degree of dehydration which is not always easy to assess on clinical examination. At the same time it would be appropriate to group and cross match blood. An X-ray of the abdomen in both supine and erect positions will reveal fluid levels throughout the small gut if an obstruction is present in the large bowel, which is likely in this case. In addition a proctoscopy and sigmoidoscopy must be performed and faecal matter tested for occult blood. These investigations may reveal the nature and site of an obstruction in the rectum or sigmoid colon. If a pathological lesion is seen, biopsies should be taken.

In the presence of intestinal obstruction the fluid balance status initially determines your management. Where considerable fluid loss and dehydration exist, the patient must have intravenous fluid (and calorific) replacement. With persistent vomiting nasogastric suction should be instituted. Fluid depletion must be corrected prior to any surgical procedure. Conservative treatment may be attempted, however if severe pain persists and signs of obstruction remain, then laparotomy is indicated.

The most likely diagnosis is that of a carcinoma of the colon or rectum. However other malignancies may exert external pressure on the lower bowel and present in this way. Constipation without any underlying pathology may present as acute intestinal obstruction and should always be considered.

Diverticulosis associated with alteration in bowel habit characterised by alternating periods of diarrhoea and constipation is a less likely possibility.

45

A 19 year old unemployed typist had been married for two years but had separated from her husband 9 months previously. She had no significant past history except that both her mother and father were twins and her maternal grandmother had given birth to triplets. Her first pregnancy, shortly after her marriage, ended with a low forceps delivery of a live female infant which weighed 3.65 kg.

During her first attendance at the antenatal clinic in her second pregnancy the uterine size was equivalent to 18 weeks of amenorrhoea. As she had, however, become pregnant immediately after stopping oral contraception, ultrasound cephalometry was performed which confirmed the duration of gestation. She attended the antenatal clinic regularly and no complications were detected apart from slightly excessive weight gain. During her last visit to the clinic at 39 weeks the fetal and uterine size corresponded to term. The lie was longitudinal with a cephalic presentation. The head was engaged when the patient was sitting up and the position was thought to be occipito-posterior.

Labour commenced four days later and at the time of admission she was having strong contractions every two to three minutes. Her membranes had ruptured an hour earlier and clear amniotic fluid was draining. The abdominal findings were unchanged and the fetal heart rate was 150 beats per minute. Vaginal examination revealed that the position was right occipito-posterior and that the cervix was four centimetres dilated and fully effaced. Despite good contractions progress was relatively slow and she only became fully dilated ten hours later. At this time the head was still right occipito-posterior and just above the level of the ischial spines. Maternal effort was good during the second stage but after half an hour the head was still not visible. A further vaginal examination revealed that the head was now level with the ischial spines and right occipito-transverse. There was a moderate caput but minimal moulding and although the ischial spines were rather prominent, the dimensions of the pelvic outlet were thought to be adequate for a vaginal delivery.

1. What is the diagnosis and what is the aetiology of this condition?
2. Describe three methods for managing this complication of labour.

This patient has a 'deep transverse arrest'. This results from the failure of the fetal head to rotate completely from the occipito-posterior position to the occipito-anterior, and the consequent arrest of descent at the level of the ischial spines. This failure of rotation is usually due to deficient flexion of the head and it probably also accounts for the occipito-posterior position at the onset of labour. For a head in the occipito-posterior position to become occipito-anterior it has to rotate through three eighths of a circle. If the pelvis is slightly narrow or the ischial spines prominent then this may prevent rotation beyond the transverse position.

When this complication arises an assisted delivery is necessary. The head must first be rotated to the occipito-anterior position and this is usually performed with rotation forceps, of which Kielland's are the most popular variety. Alternatively a hand can be introduced into the vagina and the fetal head rotated manually. Both of these procedures are painful and require either general anaesthesia or fully effective epidural analgesia.

After rotation with Kielland's forceps an episiotomy is performed and the head is then delivered by downward and backward traction on the forceps. Following manual rotation it is usual to apply curved foceps such as Simpson's or Anderson's to the head and after an episiotomy to effect delivery by traction along the pelvic axis.

Some obstetricians prefer to remove the Kielland's forceps after successful rotation and complete the delivery with curved forceps to minimise perineal trauma. The vacuum extractor (Ventouse) may also be used to effect rotation and delivery. The largest cup that can be applied is attached as close to the occiput as possible. Once a vacuum of $0.8 \, kg/cm^2$ has been achieved traction is applied both to encourage flexion and draw the head downwards. The protagonists of this method claim that rotation then occurs at the 'appropriate' level which may even be at the perineum. When performed correctly it requires minimal anaesthesia, often only perineal infiltration or at most a pudendal block. It is important to stress that these three methods of delivery, unlike simple forceps, all require considerably more skill and experience than is required for mid-cavity or outlet forceps.

46

A 68 year old man was admitted to hospital with a one week history of bruising. He denied any history of trauma and stated that he had always been in excellent health.

On examination, generalised purpura and petichiae were evident over the trunk and limbs and a haemorrhagic lesion was present on his tongue. No enlarged lymph nodes were palpable and the abdominal examination revealed no visceromegaly. Examination of the cardiovascular and respiratory systems was normal except that on fundoscopy several small haemorrhages were present in both retinae.

Initial investigations: Hb 12 g/dl; WBC 6 x 10^9/l; platelets 8 x 10^9/l. Blood urea and electrolytes normal. Chest X-ray normal.

1. Give a differential diagnosis of this man's illness.
2. What investigations would be most likely to establish a diagnosis and what features should be identified?

This elderly man has a haemorrhagic disorder which is associated with thrombocytopenia and for which there are many possible causes. These may be classified as those disorders in which there is decreased production of platelets and those in which the platelets are destroyed.

In the former category the following must be considered:— replacement of bone marrow by leukaemia or other malignant process (including myelofibrosis); aplasia due to toxins, e.g. drugs, chemicals or irradiation; splenomegaly due to any cause; certain bacterial and viral infections and occasionally in deficiency disorders, e.g. vitamin B_{12} and vitamin C deficiency.

Increased destruction of platelets occurs in idiopathic thrombocytopenic purpura; as a result of autoantibodies produced in response to certain drugs (e.g. sulphonamides, sedormid, P.A.S.) or in association with lupus erythematosus, glandular fever, and some carcinomas and leukaemias; and as a consequence of severe infections and disseminated intravascular coagulation.

In the absence of a history of drug ingestion, recent infection or other illness many of these diagnoses are less probable and the likely diagnosis is that of idiopathic thrombocytopenic purpura (ITP) or a leukaemia (despite the normal Hb and WBC).

The diagnosis is best confirmed by performing a bone marrow examination. In ITP megakaryocytes are abundant and immature forms present. Precursors of the other blood forming cells are normal in contrast to leukaemia or bone marrow infiltration by tumour.

47

Two patients presented complaining of double vision.

The first was a 25 year old cobbler. He found that when reaching to the left for his hammer he saw two hammers. His wife then told him that his face was 'not right'. The second, a 23 year old physiology student on holiday from his native Germany, found he was seeing double while trying to drive.

On examination, the cobbler had weakness of the muscles of expression of the whole of the left side of his face, including the muscles of the forehead. The only abnormality of ocular movements was a failure of the left eye to abduct when attempting to look to the left. The student had no facial weakness. When he attempted to look to the left his right eye failed to adduct, and although the left eye abducted, it showed a coarse nystagmus when abducted. When he looked to the right there was no abnormality in the movement of the left eye, but the right eye failed to abduct.

Both men had absent abdominal reflexes. There were no other abnormal physical signs. The patients did not seem particularly concerned about their symptoms, which gradually improved over the next few weeks. Both suffered relapses in the next few months.

1. Where are the lesions causing diplopia in the two men?
2. Both suffered from the same disease: what was it?
3. What is the prognosis?

Diagnosis of lesions of this type is an exercise in simple applied neuroanatomy, and there is no substitute for an adequate knowledge of the structure of the nervous system.

The cobbler has a left sixth cranial nerve palsy and a left seventh nerve palsy of lower motor neurone type. These can easily be explained by a single lesion at the nucleus of the sixth nerve which is, of course, in direct relation with the genu of the facial nerve. In the case of the student, the combination of inability to adduct the right eye with coarse nystagmus of the left eye on abduction shows that there is a lesion of the right medial longitudinal fasciculus (which coordinates conjugate movements of the eyes to the left) producing an internuclear ophthalmoplegia. The presence of inability to abduct the right eye, a sixth nerve palsy, shows that the lesion is at the posterior end of the medial longitudinal fasciculus where it passes close to the right abducent (sixth nerve) nucleus.

The localised cerebral lesions with a tendency to relapse and remit in young people are highly suggestive of disseminated sclerosis. This diagnosis is supported by the absent abdominal reflexes, a common early sign in this disease, and by the characteristic and curious indifference to disability shown by the two men: although some neurologists deny that this 'Belle indifference' is peculiar to demyelinating disease.

The prognosis in disseminated sclerosis is variable, unpredictable and often less gloomy than supposed. A small minority of patients show a rapid downhill course: most have repeated relapses and remissions with a gradual decline over many years into chronic disability. A reasonable number of patients have one or two acute episodes of illness but then seem to remain in good health for many years. It is impossible to say how many fall into this group as many cases may remain undiagnosed.

48

You are doing a locum for the house physician who is on holiday, and the ward staff nurse calls to say that she is worried about a patient admitted two hours previously after taking an overdose of morphine and alcohol. She was semiconscious on admission and had been 'washed out' in casualty. On arrival to the ward she was drowsy but is now unconscious with stertorous respirations.

1. Give three possible causes for the patient's deterioration.
2. How may your physical examination assist in making a diagnosis?
3. Give three important investigations.
4. Outline your principles for management of the problem.

Self poisoning with drugs at present constitutes one of the commonest causes of admission to hospital. In many cases the drug of misuse or abuse is known, however, self poisoning with several agents is common and can complicate management. Respiratory depression will follow an overdose of opiates or alcohol and may alone account for the deterioration in the condition of this patient. (Note the pin-point pupils that occur with opiates). Nevertheless one must never assume that the overdose is the sole clinical insult with which you may have to deal. Head injuries are often missed in comatose patients (epileptics, diabetics, alcoholics etc.) and must be carefully looked for. Gastric lavage is a procedure which must be undertaken with great care. In any patient semiconscious or unconscious it is mandatory to perform this task after intubation to prevent the aspiration of fluid into the lungs. Where alcohol has been abused aspiration may occur prior to hospital admission. Thus an aspiration pneumonia should be considered as a possible cause of this patient's collapse.

It is important, therefore, to look for the clinical signs of head injury including local examination of the head and neck and a careful neurological examination for localising signs. Examination of the chest must be performed and scattered crepitations may provide evidence for aspiration.

When respiratory distress is encountered in an unconscious patient, assisted ventilation must be initiated following the measurement of arterial blood gases. A skull X-ray must be performed for evidence of head injury and a chest X-ray may reveal an aspiration pneumonia.

The principles for management include the assessment of severity of respiratory and cardiac function with assisted ventilation for respiratory depression in this patient.

In the case of aspiration pneumonia therapy should be directed to providing adequate oxygenation of the patient, and most physicians would administer antibiotics and steroids in an attempt to reduce the intra-alveolar oedema.

If a head injury is found a neurosurgical opinion must be sought immediately.

49

An unmarried 16 year old schoolgirl went on holiday to Amsterdam with other young friends. She returned with a sore throat and also complained to her general practitioner of 'feeling shivery' and generally unwell. She was prescribed oral ampicillin, 500 mg four times a day, and after two days developed a generalised rash. She was still unwell after five days and the antibiotic was changed to cephalexin 500 mg four times a day, orally. After a further three days she developed generalised lower abdominal pain and was sent by her general practitioner to the accident and emergency department of her local hospital.

On examination, she was afebrile but had rebound tenderness and guarding over the whole abdomen. She was admitted to the surgical ward. The cephalexin was continued. At no time was a vaginal examination performed. After seven days in hospital she remained unwell. Erect and supine X-rays of the abdomen were normal but her erythrocyte sedimentation rate was persistently above 80 mm per hour. At this point, a gynaecological opinion was sought. The menstrual history was normal, with the last period three weeks previously. On pelvic examination she had an ill-defined mass in the right adnexum, about 6 cm. in diameter. The mass was tender on palpation, as was the left adnexum although no masses were palpable on this side. The uterus appeared to be of normal size but there was considerable excitation pain on movement of the cervix.

1. What is the diagnosis?
2. What are the two most important investigations to confirm it?
3. What is the further management?
4. What is the long term prognosis?

The general practitioner assumed the girl had infectious mononucleosis after she had developed a rash on ampicillin. However, the appearance of abdominal pain following the sore throat coupled with the fact that she had been on an unsupervised holiday to Amsterdam should have suggested the possibility of gonorrhoea. The increasing prevalence of orogenital sex has meant that Neisseria gonorrhoea can be cultured from the throats of up to 10 per cent of patients with sexually transmitted disease. The patient, when questioned tactfully, did indeed give a history of several unguarded acts of sexual intercourse with casual acquaintances while on holiday. It is regrettable that a pelvic examination was not performed earlier, since the adnexal mass plus bilateral tenderness would have suggested a pelvic infection. The rash may have been due to gonococcal septicaemia, but was probably just an allergic reaction to the ampicillin.

The diagnosis was confirmed with cervical, urethral and rectal swabs which on culture all grew Neisseria gonorrhoeae, resistant to penicillin and cephaloridine. The right adnexal mass was identified as a psyosalpinx using laparoscopy. This also revealed evidence of widespread pelvic inflammation including the left tube.

The normal treatment of gonorrhoea is the intramuscular injection of 4.8 megaunits of procaine penicillin, or three grams of oral ampicillin with one gram of probenecid. Alternatively, a loading dose of one gram of a cephalosporin can be given, followed by 500mg four times daily for at least four days. An important feature of these regimes is that they are also adequate for the treatment of syphilis, which may be contracted at the same time as the gonorrhoea. Inadequate antibiotic dosage may suppress but not eradicate syphilis with the result that although tests such as the Wasserman reaction will be negative, a later recrudescence of the disease will occur with unfortunate results. Treatment with antibiotics such as co-trimoxazole or tetracycline will not normally be adequate for the spirochaete, and if as in this case antibiotic resistance necessitates their use, careful follow up of syphilitic serology is mandatory. Recent sexual contacts should also be traced where possible and offered diagnostic screening, and treatment where necessary.

Following an acute attack of pelvic sepsis requiring admission to hospital, about 30 per cent of patients have recurrent infections requiring further antibiotic therapy and about 20 per cent become sterile. The results of surgery on the damaged tubes are poor with only about a 10 per cent chance of restoring function. In a case with a proven pyosalpinx and subsequent bilateral hydrosalpinges, the likelihood of permanent sterility is about 80 per cent.

50

A 69 year old widow lived alone in a council flat. Her husband had died at the age of 49 from 'dementia'. She had attended a hypertension clinic for many years, and was taking propranolol 160 mg. b.d. and hydrochlorothiazide 50 mg daily. The dose or propranolol had recently been increased from 80 mg b.d.

She was brought to the hospital by her son, who had visited her and thought she seemed unwell. She denied that she was at all ill, and said that the only problem was that her flat was unsuitable; she explained that she was upset by the rats that ran all over her budgerigar's cage, and that the man in the flat above had started watching her undress through a magic ray in the light-fitting in her bedroom. The son confirmed that there were no rats in the flat.

On examination there were no abnormal physical signs, apart from an area of old choroido-retinitis in the right fundus. The blood pressure was 150/85 mmHg. She showed no signs of being depressed.

1. Suggest four possible causes for her mental state.
2. Give six potentially useful investigations.

While a paranoid psychosis may sometimes arise in a patient of late middle age with no apparent cause — a condition sometimes called paraphrenia, paranoid schizophrenia of late onset, and characteristically associated with no gross abnormality of affect — it is important to exclude a remediable cause for her illness. A possibility, in view of her choroidoretinitis and her husband's unusual final illness, is tertiary syphilis.

There are many other possible causes of an organic psychosis of this type, although there are no features to point to any one of them in this case. These include various infections, metabolic and endocrine conditions, as well as vitamin deficiencies and structural disorders of the brain itself. Amongst space-occupying lesions of the brain one must not forget a subdural haematoma, which very rarely presents with a psychiatric illness, sometimes without a history of injury.

Drugs can cause psychoses, especially ethanol, amphetamines and cannabis. Psychiatric disturbances are a recognised complication of treatment with propranolol.

Investigations should include a WR and fluorescent treponemal antibody tests. These should also be done on c.s.f. obtained by lumbar puncture. Other blood investigations should include a blood count and measurement of the serum vitamin B_{12} (the latter may be superfluous if the MCV is normal), and estimation of blood sugar and serum calcium. X-rays of skull and chest should be taken, and an isotope brain scan and electroencephalogram are needed to show any cerebral lesion. Specialised neuroradiology or computerised axial tomography would be indicated if a space-occupying lesion was still suspected after these simpler tests.

The WR was positive, and the patient had suffered from active syphilis in the past, although this had been treated adequately with penicillin. The psychosis was due to propranolol, and was cured by reducing the dose to 40 mg b.d., adding hydralazine to the treatment. An attempt to return to higher doses of propranolol led to a relapse of her psychosis.

51

A 55 year old publican presented with a two week history of anorexia and headache followed by a haematemesis and melaena on the day of admission to hospital. Three months prior to his admission he had started to experience vague abdominal discomfort after meals, which was associated with nausea. He admitted to having lost 7 kg in weight over this period.

On examination he was distressed, pale and sweating profusely. No enlarged lymph nodes were palpable. The pulse was 120/min, regular and BP 90/60 mmHg. The other positive findings were epigastric tenderness and fresh blood on rectal examination.

1. Suggest three possible diagnoses.
2. What precipitating factor(s) may have led to his haematemesis?
3. Outline your urgent management of this case.
4. What essential investigations would you perform?

This man presents with his first haematemesis following a three month history of gastrointestinal symptoms related to food. Peptic ulceration is a probable cause of his bleeding. However, the presence of weight loss in a man of this age raises the possibility of a gastric carcinoma. Alcoholism is common amongst publicans and bleeding oesophageal varices should always be considered. The absence of other stigmata of chronic liver disease make this less probable.

It is common for gastric bleeding to be precipitated by aspirin containing compounds and since the majority of people take mild analgesics for headaches a history of drug ingestion is important to elicit. Alcohol may produce a gastritis which may be associated with haemorrhage.

This patient is shocked (pale, sweating, tachycardia, hypotension) and requires urgent transfusion. Blood must be taken immediately for grouping and in the initial period at least 4 pints of blood should be cross matched. At the same time a haemoglobin and PCV should be obtained as a guide to the extent of previous blood loss. Note that with an acute bleed, some time may elapse before haemodilution occurs due to transfer of extracellular fluid into the vascular compartment. Thus initial haemoglobin values may appear normal.

Blood urea and electrolyte values are mandatory since intravenous fluid or blood will be required and an early estimation of the state of hydration is vital. (Elevation of the blood urea may reflect a rise in blood nitrogen from absorption and breakdown of blood from the gut. Thus careful monitoring of urine flow is required to ascertain whether renal function had been compromised by hypovolaemia). Liver function tests may be taken at the time of initial blood sampling.

An intravenous infusion should be established to counteract the fluid loss. Plasma and blood when available should be given at a rate to restore the blood volume to normal. This is monitored by recordings of central venous pressure (ideally CVP line) and arterial pressure. (Further blood loss is indicated by a fall in CVP and blood pressure).

When further haemorrhage occurs and the circulatory state cannot be controlled by transfusion, laparotomy is indicated.

The important diagnostic investigations are those of gastroscopy and biopsy where appropriate followed by barium swallow and meal.

52

A 30 year old English housewife first attended the gynaecology clinic complaining of primary infertility of five years duration. She was fully investigated and found to have anovulatory menstrual cycles but was otherwise normal. She was treated with clomiphene 50 mg daily from the fifth to the tenth day of the menstrual cycle. This did not induce ovulation and the dose was therefore increased after three months to 100 mg daily. A pregnancy resulted after the sixth course of clomiphene.

Apart from nausea and occasional vomiting the pregnancy progressed normally until 13 weeks when she was admitted as an emergency complaining of a red-brown vaginal discharge for two days. During the morning of the day of admission she experienced heavy vaginal bleeding and suprapubic cramps.

On examination her breasts were normal and active. The uterine size was equivalent to a pregnancy of 18 weeks duration, which was considerably larger than her dates suggested it should be. There was no uterine tenderness but the fetal heart could not be heard with doppler ultrasound. A speculum examination revealed approximately 250 ml of blood clot within the vagina and when this was removed the cervix was found to be approximately 2 centimetres dilated with numerous grape-like vesicles protruding through the cervical canal.

1. What is the diagnosis?
2. What investigations could be used to confirm it?
3. How would you treat this patient?
4. What advice would you give regarding future pregnancies?

This patient displayed several features suggestive of a hydatidiform (vesicular) mole, a diagnosis which should always be borne in mind when fetal heart sounds cannot be detected in a patient who has persisting pregnancy symptoms and a uterus which is large for dates. Excessive uterine enlargement, however, only occurs in about a half of the women with this condition and most present as a threatened or inevitable abortion. Expulsion of vesicular tissue which occurs sooner or later, however, makes the diagnosis obvious. Other symptoms and signs which frequently occur in these patients include excessive vomiting, anaemia, pre-eclampsia and cystic ovarian enlargement.

The disease is relatively uncommon in European communities (1 : 2,500 deliveries) but occurs in approximately one in 600 oriental women and is much more frequent over the age of 40 years.

When the diagnosis is in doubt two investigations may be used to provide confirmatory evidence. These are quantitative or semi-quantitative urinary human chorionic gonadotrophin (HCG) estimation and ultrasound scanning. The former relies on the fact that molar tissue secretes very large quantities of HCG and produces an immunological pregnancy test which is positive in a dilution of at least one in 200. Sonar produces a unique 'snow storm' picture due to the multiple echoes which arise from the cystic villi.

Evacuation of the uterus may be achieved by inducing abortion with an intravenous syntocinon or prostaglandin infusion. Alternatively, the mole may be sucked out with the apparatus used for termination of pregnancy. If an oxytocic is used to induce abortion, vacuum or simple curettage must subsequently be performed to ensure that the uterus is empty. Severe haemorrhage is a major hazard at the time of abortion and adequate blood should always be cross matched for these patients.

Choriocarcinoma follows hydatiform mole in approximately two per cent of cases and is more common in women over 40 years of age. Hysterectomy is, therefore, sometimes recommended in older women or those who have completed their family. Because it may lead to choriocarcinoma this disease should always be regarded as potentially malignant and all patients must be followed closely for two years after evacuation of the uterus in order to detect the first sign of a recurrence of chorionic activity. This involves regular measurement of HCG, so the patient must be advised to avoid becoming pregnant during this period of time.

53

A 55 year old chauffeur was dismissed after only one day with a new employer for being drunk at work. He presented to his doctor saying that he was ill and not inebriated.

The history was that for six months he had noticed gradually worsening ringing in his left ear. On several occasions he had suddenly felt that the world was spinning round and immediately lost his balance and fell to the ground.

On examination the only abnormal sign was partial deafness of the left ear. Rinne's test at the left ear was normal, and Weber's test showed that the sound of the tuning fork seemed to be coming into the right ear.

1. What is the diagnosis?
2. If the vertigo had been continuous and progressive rather than episodic, what would you suspect?
3. What treatment would you offer this man?

The history is typical of Meniere's syndrome or paroxysmal labyrinthine vertigo. This diagnosis is supported by the sign of partial deafness in the affected ear, the tests showing that the deafness is of nerve or perceptive type.

Progressive tinnitus, vertigo and deafness would be a more sinister history, suggesting a gradually developing lesion involving the eighth or acoustic nerve. Possible pathologies include a tumour such as an acoustic neuroma, chronic infection — tuberculous meningitis or rarely syphilis — or degenerative conditions involving the eighth nerve or its central connections.

Treatment of Meniere's syndrome is unsatisfactory: the most useful drugs are antiemetics, for example prochlorperazine. Simple sedatives are sometimes found to be of value. This chauffeur should consider changing his job in case disabling vertigo develops suddenly while driving.

54

A boy of 15 years was seen by his general practitioner because he had complained for two days of fever, malaise and an increasingly severe headache. A diagnosis of 'influenza' was made and he was prescribed paracetamol tablets. During the next 48 hours his condition deteriorated and he became drowsy and disorientated. He vomited several times small quantities of clear fluid.

On referral to the local hospital, he was observed to be pyrexial (39.5°) and was delirious. A macular rash was present on the trunk and purpura were noted on the arms and legs. The pulse rate was 130/min, sinus rhythm, BP 90/60 mmHg. The heart and lungs were clinically normal. No abnormalities were found on abdominal examination, but on examination of the central nervous system there was neck stiffness and papilloedema.

Initial investigations in the casualty department revealed: Hb 13.5 g/dl, WBC 30 x 10^9/l, (polymorphs 28 x 10^9/l), platelets 10 x 10^9/l. Chest X-ray and skull X-ray normal.

1. What is the most likely diagnosis, and what complication is present?
2. The casualty officer suggests that a lumbar puncture be performed. Why would you carry out this investigation and what abnormalities might be discovered?
3. What further investigations are indicated?
4. What specific therapy would you initiate for the infection?

The presenting symptoms and signs of this boy's illness suggest an infection and, in view of the abnormalities discovered on examination of the central nervous system, the diagnosis of meningitis is highly probable. This diagnosis constitutes a medical emergency and urgent investigation with the institution of appropriate therapy is required to prevent irreparable brain damage. The polymorphonuclear leucocytosis and the clinical signs of bruising with a reduced platelet count indicate a bacterial meningitis complicated by an haemorrhagic diathesis. Meningococcal septicaemia is not uncommonly associated with disseminated intravascular coagulation but this may be found in septicaemia due to any cause, and carries a poor prognosis. Haemorrhage into the adrenal glands is a particularly dangerous sequela.

If a diagnosis of meningitis is suspected a lumbar puncture must be performed. Although bacterial meningitis is suspected, it is important to isolate the causative agent (meningococcus, haemophilus influenzae or pneumococcus being most likely in this case). Viral meningitides and tuberculous meningitis may present with similar features, thus examination of the c.s.f. is mandatory.

In bacterial infections the following abnormalities will be noted in the c.s.f:— pressure raised; cells (neutrophils) increased; sugar low, protein increased. In addition, a gram stain will often reveal the causative organism, nevertheless, a culture must be arranged.

In view of the presence of purpura in association with thrombocytopenia, the diagnosis of disseminated intravascular coagulation must be confirmed by further clotting studies and estimations of plasma fibrinogen and fibrin degradation products.

Penicillin and chloramphenicol or high dose intravenous ampicillin are the most effective agents and cover infection to all three bacilli.

55

You are the locum house surgeon, and your registrar telephones you from the outpatient clinic to say that he is admitting a 48 year old man for orchidectomy for a malignant neoplasm of the testis on the next day's list.

When the patient arrives on the ward, you find on examination that one testis is replaced by a firm irregular swelling 8 x 5 x 5 cm, which appears to have arisen from the posterior aspect of the testis. In three places the mass has ulcerated through the scrotal skin, and these ulcers are discharging thick white greasy matter. There are no other abnormal signs on examination, including rectal examination.

1. Give an alternative diagnosis that must be considered.
2. What four investigations would you order at once?
3. What is the initial treatment if this is not a neoplasm?

The important alternative diagnosis is of tuberculous epididymitis. The mass appears to have arisen posteriorly in the testis, where the epididymis lies. Both tumours and tuberculous masses can ulcerate the scrotum, but the discharge of a white greasy substance suggests a tuberculous sinus leaking caseous tuberculous pus. The other mass that can ulcerate the scrotum is a gumma, but gummata are exceedingly rare, arise in the testis proper, and tend not to be irregular. The normal findings on rectal examination are relevant: tuberculous seminal vesicles can sometimes be palpated.

A Ziehl-Nielsen stained smear of the discharge should be examined, and the material sent for T.B. culture. At least 3 early morning specimens of urine should also be examined and cultured, as tuberculous epididymitis is very often associated with tuberculosis elsewhere in the urinary tract. For this reason, a plain X-ray of the abdomen and an intravenous pyelogram should be taken and examined carefully, looking particularly for calcification in the kidney and ureter on the same side as the affected epididymis. The chest must be X-rayed: active tuberculosis may be present, otherwise an old focus of infection will almost certainly be found. An ESR may be useful as a baseline in assessing the response to treatment. Biochemical tests of renal function should be done, not least in case streptomycin is included in the treatment: renal impairment potentiates the ototoxicity of aminoglycoside antibiotics which are excreted by the kidneys.

The initial treatment of epididymitis would certainly be medical. The combination of drugs chosen would have to be adjusted in the light of antibiotic sensitivity testing, but a reasonable initial choice might be rifampicin and isoniazid. The need for later surgical excision of the affected part would have to be assessed after the response to antituberculous chemotherapy could be seen.

56

A 45 year old Sri Lankan doctor's wife in her fourth pregnancy entered the country and booked for antenatal care 36 weeks after her last menstrual period. This had been normal and she was certain of the date of her last period. On examination everything seemed normal except that the fetus was thought to be only about 32 weeks size. However, uterine dimensions were compatible with the dates. A fluid thrill was palpable. Routine tests were also normal except that her haemoglobin was only 10.7 g/dl. Three weeks later her uterine size was consistent with 39 weeks gestation but an ultrasound examination showed the biparietal diameter of the fetus to be on the mean for 33 weeks. At this time a twenty four hour total oestrogen urinary excretion was 250 μmol/l. (At the laboratory in question, the mean value for thirty six weeks was 140 μmol/l with an upper tenth percentile of 240 μmol/l). Two weeks later, at term plus five days by dates, the lie of the fetus had become transverse and the patient was admitted for investigation.

1. What diagnoses would you consider?
2. What investigations would you perform?
3. Outline your further management.

This woman had a fetus which was apparently small for dates. However, dysmaturity is usually associated with oligohydramnios and this patient had a fluid thrill which indicated excess liquor. In addition the oestrogen excretion was above the normal upper limit for a singleton whereas a dysmature infant is normally associated with a reduced value. The fetal lie was unstable and the patient was anaemic. All of these features should suggest the possibility of a multiple pregnancy. Ultrasound is normally a useful diagnostic tool in this situation but like any procedure which relies heavily on human expertise, its use is subject to human error. One must also consider the possibility of mistaken dates on the part of the patient, particularly in one who books late. If we assume that the woman conceived four weeks later than she thought, then the gestation of the fetus was compatible with clinical and ultrasound estimation of its size, and the problem is converted to one of a large-for-dates uterus with excess liquor. This could simply have been due to hydramnios, but the anaemia and high oestrogen are more in favour of multiple pregnancy.

The best diagnostic procedure in this situation is an oblique X-ray of the abdomen. This might have revealed fetal abnormalities, accounting for the hydramnios but in fact confirmed the clinical suspicion of twins.

In view of the obvious uncertainty about the gestation, the pregnancy was allowed to continue, with monitoring of oestrogen excretion, biparietal diameter growth and daily cardiotocographic tracing of the fetal heart. (When the gestation is certain, twins are often induced at term because failure of placental function and fetal growth occurs about two weeks earlier than in singletons.)

Spontaneous onset of labour occurred at 44 weeks by dates. Labour and delivery were uneventful, Gestational assessment of the neonates suggested that they were at term. They weighed 2.13 kg and 2.21 kg, which is small by singleton standards but less unusual for twins.

57

A 54 year old housewife complained of tiredness and shortness of breath. On closer questioning she said that she found that mild exertion such as carrying a little shopping on the flat made her exhausted, and the shortness of breath was worse when lying flat. The only past history of note was an episode of St Vitus Dance at the age of twelve. She was nulliparous.

On examination, the temperature was 37.6°C and the pulse was regular. The first heart sound was loud, and there was a harsh pansystolic murmur at the apex radiating to the axilla. There was no third heart sound and some experienced observers could hear a soft low-pitched diastolic murmur at the apex. There were crepitations at the lung bases, and the jugular venous pressure was elevated to four centimetres above the sternal edge. There was slight ankle oedema and one ankle joint was red, swollen and very tender.

1. What is your interpretation of the signs in the heart?
2. Give two important causes of the signs at the ankle, and indicate other possible diagnoses of the arthropathy.

Following prolonged treatment in hospital with bed rest, digoxin and diuretics she was discharged with the shortness of breath much improved, but still very tired. At her first out-patient visit she complained of the sudden onset of pain in the right side of the chest, the pain being made worse by breathing. On examination, a rub was audible at the site of maximum pain, but the heart murmurs had disappeared. She was readmitted, and a few days later a letter arrived from her general practitioner saying that while he was grateful for all the attention she had received, he had hoped a few weeks before her first admission that she would be seen by a rheumatologist, as she had been unwell with an arthritis of rheumatoid type, associated with a very high ESR and weakly positive rheumatoid factor tests.

3. What is the most important diagnosis to consider as a cause for her chest pain?
4. The letter from the patient's family doctor suggests a single diagnosis that would explain the history and physical signs found at both admissions. What is this diagnosis?

The pansystolic murmur described is typical of mitral regurgitation (incompetence). However, uncomplicated mitral incompetence is associated with a soft first heart sound (due to failure of the mitral valve cusps to meet as the valve closes) and there is often a third heart sound as the overfilled left atrium empties into the ventricle. The loud first sound is evidence that mitral stenosis is present in addition to the incompetence, and the diastolic murmur that some can hear confirms this. The history of chorea points to rheumatic mitral valve disease.

The monoarticular arthritis could be due to gout, which is always an important diagnosis, especially in patients who are likely to need treatment with thiazide diuretics. Bacterial endocarditis can cause an arthropathy, and could also explain the symptom of tiredness (which, however, could be due to cardiac failure alone) and the fever. A careful search for other signs that might be explained by endocarditis should be made. Acute bacterial arthritis often involves one joint only, but any of the many diseases that usually cause a polyarthropathy can present in a single joint.

The sudden onset of pleuritic pain, particularly in a patient who has been resting in bed, suggests a pulmonary embolus. She was investigated with this diagnosis in mind.

The diagnosis suggested by the additional history from the general practitioner is systemic lupus erythematosus. This would explain the tiredness, fever, arthritis, pleurisy and the laboratory findings, all these being typical of SLE. The commonest cardiac manifestation of SLE is pericarditis, but an endocarditis — Libman-Sacks endocarditis — can occur and can cause evanescent mitral valve lesions. If the diagnosis of SLE were not confirmed, the change in the heart murmurs would be strongly in favour of bacterial endocarditis.

58

You are the house surgeon, and are covering emergencies for a number of your colleagues. The night sister asks you to see a patient who is confused. You have not met him before.

You find from the notes that he is a 42 year old doctor who has cirrhosis of the liver secondary to viral hepatitis that he caught as a student. He has had a number of haematemeses from his oesophageal varices, and 5 days previously had an emergency side-to-side portacaval anastomosis to control torrential gastrointestinal haemorrhage. The only treatment since operation has been papaveretum 10 mg p.r.n. for pain, twice daily colonic washouts, and 5 per cent dextrose 500 ml 8 hourly intravenously, each 500 ml supplemented with 20 mmol potassium chloride. He has been allowed sips of water by mouth, but no other fluids or food.

1. What are likely causes of confusion in such a patient?
2. Following your examination of the patient, you arrange a number of investigations. The first results show: plasma sodium 108 mmol/l, potassium 3.4 mmol/l, urea 2.3 mmol/l (normal 2.5 — 6.6 mmol/l); urine sodium 2 mmol/l, potassium 32 mmol/l (the urine estimations being carried out on a single sample of urine passed at the time of your examination). What do you suspect?

In patients after operation, the causes of any complication should be considered in a logical scheme: problems peculiar to the operation performed, problems common to all operations; problems classified by the likely pathology, and problems classified by the system of the body involved.

In this example, there are causes of confusion common to all patients after abdominal operations and causes particular to portasystemic anastomoses. The most important of the latter is hepatic encephalopathy: this is especially common after side-to-side portacaval anastomosis rather than other forms of portasystemic shunt, and in this patient might have been precipitated by the prescription for opiate analgesia. On the other hand, he has taken no nitrogen-containing foods, and his colon has been washed out, with the aim of preventing encephalopathy. Possible pathologies causing confusion common to all patients after abdominal surgery include infection, anoxia, haemorrhage and electrolyte imbalance. Infection might be in chest, wound or abdomen; anoxia could follow pulmonary emboli, respiratory depression due to drugs, or chest infection; haemorrhage might be into the wound, at the site of operation within the abdomen, or into the gut; electrolyte disturbances might be due to acute renal failure or might be iatrogenic.

The last of these has occurred in this case. He has been given potassium and water intravenously for five days. This is enough to cause postoperative sodium deprivation, and one can see from the urine sodium concentration that the kidneys are adjusting to the body's lack of sodium by avid reabsorption of sodium from the glomerular filtrate. The sodium deficit and relative water overload may have been exacerbated by absorption of water from the gut during colonic washouts.

In this patient there were no signs of any other cause of confusion, including portasystemic encephalopathy. He improved dramatically when the fluid in the intravenous infusion was changed to 'normal' saline, 2 litres (308 mmol sodium chloride) each day.

59

A family of two adults and two children spent three weeks camping on a farm in mid-Wales. Two weeks after returning home, the 53-year old father started to complain of headaches and lethargy. These symptoms continued for four days and were associated with fever and rigors. He felt better after taking aspirin but one week later his symptoms returned and on this occasion he also experienced aches and pains in the legs and back, pain in his knee, hip and elbow joints and a non-productive cough.

His past medical history included jaundice at the age of 18 years and malaria ten years previously when working in Nigeria.

On examination he appeared unwell. He was not clinically anaemic or jaundiced but there were palpable lymph nodes in the axillae and supraclavicular fossae which were slightly tender. His temperature was 38.5°, pulse 96/min, regular and BP 110/70 mmHg. The heart and lungs were normal. In the abdomen, the spleen was palpable 3 cm below the left costal margin. Central nervous system examination was normal.

Preliminary investigations revealed Hb 13.7 g/dl; WBC 4.5 x 10^9/l, (neutrophils 2.5 10^9/l, lymphocytes 2 x 10^9/l); ESR 50 mm/h. The chest X-ray was within normal limits.

1. Give a differential diagnosis for this man's presentation.
2. What further investigations are indicated?
3. What is the appropriate treatment for your most probable diagnosis?

A febrile illness associated with generalised symptoms and physical signs that include lymphadenopathy and splenomegaly may suggest a number of possible causes. However, the circumstances under which the illness may have been acquired, notably the camping holiday on a farm in Wales, raise the likelihood of exposure to brucella — transmitted by ingestion of milk from infected cows. Other conditions with a similar presentation include infectious mononucleosis, reticuloses, e.g. Hodgkin's disease and influenza, although the positive findings of lymphadenopathy and splenomegaly make the latter diagnosis less likely. Malaria must be considered, particularly in view of the history.

The neutrapenia and relative lymphocytosis are compatible with a brucella infection, and the diagnosis may be further substantiated by examination of serum for brucella agglutinins. Blood cultures are positive for brucella in approximately half the cases. Skin tests for brucella antigens are unreliable. In this case blood films must be examined for malarial parasites and if the diagnosis is not established a lymph node biopsy would be indicated.

The appropriate treatment for brucellosis is oxytetracycline. This drug should be given for a period of 2-3 weeks, as relapses are not infrequent and should be treated with a further course of this antibiotic.

60

A 30 year old primigravid South African woman first attended the antenatal clinic after 16 weeks amenorrhoea. She gave a history of rheumatic fever and jaundice in childhood but had not experienced any long term complications from these illnesses. On examination her uterine size was found to be equivalent to 16 weeks and the only abnormality detected was mild hypertension (150/90 mmHg). At subsequent antenatal visits her blood pressure was normal and her pregnancy progressed uneventfully until 36 weeks. At this visit the fetus was thought to be slightly large for dates and glycosuria (one plus on dip stick testing) was noted on routine urine examination. Because of the glycosuria an oral glucose tolerance test was arranged. When seen in the antenatal clinic the following week the patient complained that the baby had not moved for several days.

On examination the fetal heart could not be heard but no other abnormality was noted. The glucose tolerance test result was:

Fasting 5.2 mmol/l
30 minutes 9.4 mmol/l
60 minutes 9.8 mmol/l
90 minutes 9.0 mmol/l
120 minutes 8.1 mmol/l
150 minutes 6.2 mmol/l
180 minutes 5.0 mmol/l

1. What is the most likely diagnosis?
2. How would you confirm this?
3. How would you manage this pregnancy?

This patient appears to have experienced an intrauterine fetal death (IUD) due to chemical diabetes, probably produced by the pregnancy. The IUD can most easily be confirmed using doppler or real time pulsed ultrasound to confirm the absence of fetal heart activity. If these facilities are not available an oblique abdominal X-ray should be obtained. Early radiographic signs of fetal death are gas in the heart and major vessels together with hyperflexion of the fetal spine; later the skull bones overlap (Spalding's sign). Twenty four hour urine oestriol excretion falls to a very low level immediately after fetal death and this investigation may therefore provide additional evidence.

Patients with an IUD eventually go into spontaneous labour and there is no immediate danger to the patient if an expectant policy is adopted. The risk of disseminated intravascular coagulation and resulting hypofibrinogenaemia does not arise until three to four weeks have elapsed. It is, however, often preferable to induce labour because of the psychological effects on the mother who has to carry a dead baby.

Surgical methods of induction are contraindicated because of the risk of intrauterine infection and it is therefore usual to induce labour with intravenous oxytocin infusion or prostaglandins if this fails. High dose oxytocin therapy is frequently necessary and as this has a marked antidiuretic effect it is best given using an infusion pump which avoids the administration of large volumes of fluid and possible 'water intoxication' leading to fits.

61

A 53 year old American was on holiday in England. Her husband phoned the hotel doctor at 3.00 a.m. saying that she had woken up distressed and short of breath. On the previous evening they had attended a family reunion and had returned to their hotel uneventfully.

She had previously been in very good health except for a history of epilepsy since childhood for which she took daily phenytoin and phenobarbitone. The last fit was six months previously. There was a strong family history of ischaemic heart disease.

On examination she was apyrexial, severely distressed, tachypnoeic and cyanosed. The pulse was 120/min regular; BP 100/70 mmHg; JVP was not elevated; no peripheral oedema. The heart sounds were normal.

In the chest, there was an equivocal decrease in the percussion note over the right lower zone. In this area bronchial breathing was audible and crepitations were present throughout both mid and lower zones. There were no abnormalities in the abdomen or c.n.s.

1. Give three possible causes for her breathlessness.
2. What pathology might account for the abnormal pulmonary signs?
3. Suggest a precipitating cause for the current illness.
4. Simple investigations e.g. chest X-ray, e.c.g. and blood gases were performed.
   What abnormality would be found on blood gas analysis?
5. Outline your immediate management.

Severe respiratory distress of acute onset in an epileptic, particularly when associated with localising signs in the chest, must alert you to the possibility of aspiration occurring during a fit. The previous evening's 'reunion' could well have provided alcohol which may precipitate fits in epileptics, and other evidence for a nocturnal fit must be sought, e.g. wet bed due to micturition during the fit or residual neurological signs (Todd's paralysis). Acute dyspnoea and cyanosis may occur in several other conditions such as pneumonia of bacterial or viral origin, a pulmonary embolus or indeed acute left ventricular failure — all possible diagnoses.

The described physical signs of dullness to percussion, bronchial breathing and crepitations are those of consolidation of the lung.

Investigations on this lady confirmed bilateral shadowing in both mid and lower zones with confluent shadows in the right lower lobe. The e.c.g. showed a tachycardia and was otherwise normal. The cyanosis was confirmed by an arterial Po_2 of 50 mmHg which was associated with a low Pco_2 (30 mmHg). Hypoxia with a low Pco_2 is found in pneumonia, pulmonary emboli and pulmonary oedema and is the result of a ventilation-perfusion imbalance.

The management of aspiration pneumonia requires urgent correction of arterial hypoxaemia by administering oxygen by mask in unrestricted concentration. If immediate improvement in arterial oxygenation is not achieved, bronchoscopy and aspiration must be performed for the possible removal of a foreign body. Subsequently the combined use of steroids and antibiotics has been advocated in aspiration pneumonia to reduce the inflammatory alveolitis and prevent secondary infection.

62

The patient, who was aged 54, lived with his father and younger brother. Their mother had died at the age of 48 of bleeding from a gastric carcinoma. The patient was brought to casualty by his father, who said he was fed up because the son was refusing to help with the family scrap metal business, and had retired to his bed for the last two weeks.

The only symptom that the patient would volunteer was lassitude. On direct questioning he admitted that he was short of breath after four or five stairs, that his feet were numb and tingling, and that he was unsteady when he walked, particularly in the dark. He did not smoke, and drank beer at the weekends only. His diet was good and varied, thanks to the family allotment. He was taking no drugs, and there were no symptoms whatever relevant to his gut. On examination, the patient was very pale, and grey-haired. His skin was slighly yellow. There was a systolic murmur at the base of the heart, and the liver was enlarged by 3 cm, smooth and slightly tender. Vibration and joint position sensation were completely lost in both feet, and the loss of vibration sensation extended up to the pelvis. The gait was ataxic and Romberg's sign was positive. Knee jerks were diminished and the ankle jerks were absent, but the plantar responses were upgoing.

A blood count showed:

Hb	4.8 g/dl
WBC	$3.6 \times 10^9/l$
Platelets	$100 \times 10^9/l$
RBC	$1.8 \times 10^{12}/l$
MCV	114 fl

1. What is the diagnosis?
2. Explain the neurological signs.
3. What three other tests would you like to confirm the diagnosis?
4. What treatment would you recommend, and how would you assess its efficacy?

The patient has a severe anaemia, and many of his symptoms and signs — lassitude, dyspnoea, cardiac murmurs — could be found in any severe anaemia. The blood picture is macrocytic, as shown by the very high MCV, and there are a number of features to suggest that the case is Addisonian pernicious anaemia. These features include the family history of gastric carcinoma (which is associated with associated with achlorhydria), yellowish skin, grey hair, hepatomegaly, symptoms and signs of subacute combined degeneration of the cord, and mildly depressed white cell and platelet counts.

Depressed tendon jerks must be due to a lower motor neurone lesion or a peripheral sensory neuropathy: upgoing toes show that there is also an upper motor neurone lesion, probably of the lateral columns of the spinal cord. The dorsal columns of the cord are also involved, with loss of vibration and joint position sensation. The ataxy of gait and Rombergism are secondary to this loss of proprioceptive sense.

Other causes of a macrocytic anaemia are very unlikely in this case. The diet is good, and probably adequate in folate, there are no symptoms of malabsorption, and no drugs that might interfere with metabolism of haemopoietic factors. Beer at weekends only could not cause a macrocytic anaemia of this severity.

A bone marrow examination will confirm megaloblastic erythropoiesis, and may be useful for comparison with any later bone marrow. Blood should be taken for assay of serum vitamin B_{12} concentration, but treatment should not await this result. A test of the absorption of radioactive vitamin B_{12} (Schilling test) will confirm the inability to absorb an oral dose of vitamin B_{12} in the absence of 'intrinsic factor', and has the added advantage that the large intramuscular dose of vitamin B_{12} used to flush the radioactive vitamin B_{12} into the urine starts the treatment of the disease.

The treatment of choice is intramuscular injections of hydroxycobalamin. There is no justification for the use of cyanocabalamin. In a patient with neurological involvement the dose chosen would be higher and given more frequently than in the uncomplicated cases of pernicious anaemia. Monthly maintenance injections of vitamin B_{12} must continue for life. The initial response to vitamin B_{12} is assessed by daily reticulocyte counts, which may rise to very high values within a week of starting treatment. In any case where there is doubt about the peripheral haematological response a second bone marrow can be compared with the pretreatment specimen, and the reversion to normoblastic erythropoiesis confirmed.

63

A 27 year old civil servant had experienced the menarche at the age of fourteen. Subsequently her periods had been light and irregular, with intervals sometimes as long as six months between each bleed. At the age of twenty she married and started taking a 30 μg oestrogen combined oral contraceptive 'pill'. She was very pleased that while taking this she had regular monthly withdrawal bleeds. After four and a half years she and her husband decided that they wished to start a family and so she discontinued the 'pill'. Unfortunately, spontaneous periods did not recommence. After nine months amenorrhoea, she visited her general practitioner who referred her to the gynaecological outpatient clinic.

1. What is her diagnosis?
2. What further symptoms should you ask about?
3. What signs may be present?
4. What is the most likely therapy?

The 'catch' here is to label the patient as having 'post pill amenorrhoea'. Unfortunately this descriptive term does not represent a real diagnosis, since the whole spectrum of causes of secondary amenorrhoea must be considered. The most likely diagnoses are hyperprolactinaemia, a defect in the hypothalamopituitary ovarian cycle mechanism (usually clomiphene responsive) or weight related amenorrhoea.

The most serious possibility is hyperprolactinaemia, since a significant number of patients with this condition have a pituitary tumour. One should therefore always ask about visual disturbances (which may indicate pressure on the optic chiasma) or symptoms of raised intracranial pressure (such as headache). In addition, some patients will have inappropriate lactation. The cycling defects are often associated with emotional disturbance, or disturbances of diurnal rhythm such as those produced by intercontinental travel. Emotional disturbances are also characteristic of the patients with weight related amenorrhoea, and this group includes all cases of anorexia nervosa. Questioning should therefore always cover the social, emotional and psychiatric history of the patient.

The most striking sign which may be found is inappropriate lactation. More commonly however signs of oestrogen deficiency will be found, namely small breasts, thin vulval skin, a dry atrophic vagina, and a small uterus and ovaries. This lack of oestrogen can be confirmed by failure of withdrawal bleeding following a course of orally administered progestogen. (Withdrawal bleeding may have occurred on the pill in this patient because of the oestrogen which the pill itself contains.) The lack of oestrogen effects is not however diagnostic of any particular cause of amenorrhoea. Signs of recent weight loss may also be present.

Rarely, other physical signs may be found on laparoscopy, notably the cystic ovaries of the Stein-Leventhal syndrome (polycystic ovary syndrome) or the small inactive ovaries of premature ovarian failure. Even rarer are visual field defects, and papilloedema due to raised intracranial pressure. Most patients will respond to treatment with clomiphene but in cases of hyperprolactinaemia the specific treatment is bromocriptine. In clomiphene resistant cases (and particularly those in the weight related group who cannot regain weight) direct induction of ovulation with human menopausal gonadotrophin (Pergonal) and human chorionic gonadotrophin (HCG) may be necessary. In women with the Stein-Leventhal syndrome androgen production is excessive. It may be reduced by suppressing the adrenal component with glucocorticoids or reducing the ovarian component by bilateral resection of a wedge of ovarian tissue.

64

Miss Jones was aged 21. She had never been ill until one summer she noticed that her urine was frothy, and that her ankles were swollen. The swelling got progressively worse, until it involved her whole body, including her face.

On admission to hospital there was gross oedema of both legs and of the skin of the abdominal and chest walls. There was also periorbital oedema. There were signs of ascites and of bilateral pleural effusions. Investigations on admission showed: plasma albumin 18 g/l (normal 35-50), globulin 31 g/l (25-30), creatinine 100 μmol/l (60-120). The urine volume was 1200 ml/d, containing 24 g/d of protein and 9.6 mmol/l of creatinine.

Large doses of diuretics were needed to clear her oedema, which eventually responded to a combination of frusemide, amiloride and hydrochlorothiazide. She soon felt well enough to sunbathe on the ward balcony, but one day developed an erythematous desquamating rash over those parts of the skin that had been exposed to the sun.

1. Explain the pathophysiology of her oedema.
2. What is the likely cause of her rash?

The nephrotic syndrome is defined as oedema due to hypoproteinaemia due to protein loss through the kidney, and is the diagnosis in this case. She has a very marked leak of protein into the urine — it caused the frothiness of her urine that she noted — and a consequent fall in plasma albumin. The modest rise in plasma globulin may be related to the immunological process attacking the glomeruli and making them leak albumin. Globulins are larger than albumin, so less likely to leak into the urine, but they are much less osmotically active than albumin and are of little use in holding fluid in the circulation. Hypoalbuminaemia causes oedema by upsetting the Starling forces in and around the capillary: the plasma oncotic pressure is insufficient to work against the hydrostatic forces for the necessary reabsorption of fluid from the interstitial space into the intravascular space. The oedema tends to collect in dependant parts, for example the ankles, or in areas where the tissues are lax and can accomodate large volumes of fluid: the orbits and serous cavities. Despite the leakage of protein, other functions of the kidney are reasonable: the creatinine clearance is only slightly reduced at 80 ml/min.

An erythematous desquamating rash in a patient with a renal problem might suggest a streptococcal infection. However, there are two arguments against this in Miss Jones' case. The first is that the rash should precede the renal problem (or at least occur simultaneously) and not vice-versa. The second is that the rash is photosensitive, unlike poststreptococcal eruptions and suggesting a drug reaction. Indeed, any unexplained rash in a patient on drugs might be due to the treatment. In this case there is an obvious culprit: hydrochlorothiazide. Thiazide sensitivity is often manifest as a rash on areas exposed to sunlight.

65

A 39 year old Pakistani housewife had been unwell for six months. She was irritable, depressed and had lost 7 kg in weight. When she visited her general practitioner she also complained of increasing shortness of breath on exertion and swelling of the ankles and lower legs.

Physical examination revealed a thin rather tense woman with a temperature of 38.5°C. The pulse was 146/min and irregular, BP 95/70 mmHg. The jugular venous pulse was elevated to the angle of the jaw and pitting oedema of the feet and lower legs was present. The heart was not clinically enlarged but the apex beat was difficult to locate and the heart sounds were soft. There were no murmurs. In the chest widespread crepitations were audible throughout both lung fields and in the abdomen the liver was enlarged and tender.

Investigations carried out by the practitioner: Hb 12 g/dl; blood urea and electrolytes normal; e.c.g. — atrial fibrillation.

1. Give two possible causes for the development of cardiac failure.
2. What other physical signs would be helpful in establishing a possible diagnosis?
3. The general practitioner treated this patient with digitalis and diuretics with little success. What essential investigations and alternative treatment would you recommend?

There are many possible causes for the progressive development of cardiac failure in a middle aged or elderly person, the commonest being ischaemic, valvular and hypertensive heart disease. The clinical features in the presentation of this patient suggest alternative possibilities, since the age and sex of the patient, the absence of heart murmurs and a low blood pressure make the former aetologies less likely.

Weight loss, irritability and an arrhythmia are features of thyrotoxicosis which could well account for this presentation. However, in this patient examination of the thyroid gland was normal, and other possible signs of thyroid disease such as exophthalmos and hyperflexia were absent. The presence of a fever in association with a chronic wasting illness in an immigrant should alert you to the diagnosis of tuberculosis which was subsequently confirmed in this patient. Gross cardiac failure in the absence of cardiomegaly suggests pericardial constriction. Commonly a rise in the jugular venous pulse on inspiration may be demonstrated, however, when the JVP is grossly elevated this may be difficult to elicit. Pulsus paradoxus (an exaggerated reduction in pulse pressure and rate during inspiration) may also be present.

Investigations must include a chest X-ray, which in addition to pulmonary oedema may reveal pericardial calcification in tuberculous pericarditis. A Mantoux test and sputum analysis for tubercle bacilli should be performed. Thyroid function tests such as a protein bound iodine, serum thyroxine, T3 resin uptake or uptake would be indicated.

The failure of this patient to respond to digitalis and diuretics is not surprising. In thyrotoxic heart disease, antithyroid drugs must be administered as soon as the diagnosis is established. Note that ß-blocking drugs must not be given to control the heart rate, since the patient is in cardiac failure. With constrictive percarditis a thoracotomy and pericardectomy should be arranged.

66

A 21 year old Greek Cypriot attended the gynaecology outpatient clinic complaining of right sided lower abdominal pain of six months duration. She had at first only experienced pain during the week before her periods but for two months it had also occurred during intercourse. Her menarche had been at the age of 13 years and she had always had a regular 28 day menstrual cycle with periods lasting for between four and five days. There was no history of post coital or intermenstrual bleeding and she did not have any abnormal vaginal discharge. She had been having regular intercourse without contraception since her marriage eighteen months previously and was most anxious to become pregnant. She had had an appendicectomy in Cyprus at the age of 17 years.

Abdominal examination revealed slight tenderness in the right iliac fossa with some guarding but no rebound tenderness. On pelvic examination she was found to have a normal sized uterus which was anteverted and mobile. A tender, soft fluctuant mass approximately 8-10 cms in diameter was felt on the right side; it was situated behind the uterus and appeared to be fixed to it. The left adnexal area was normal.

Examination under general anaesthesia confirmed these findings and at laparotomy the right ovary was found to be enlarged to form a bluish coloured cyst approximately eight centimetres in diameter which was tethered in the pouch of Douglas and to the posterior aspect of the uterus and broad ligament by fine adhesions. The uterus, left ovary and both fallopian tubes were normal, it was therefore decided to remove the ovarian cyst but during the dissection the cyst wall ruptured, spilling copious thick chocolate material into the pelvis.

1. What is the most likely diagnosis?
2. What is the aetiology of this condition?
3. How would you treat this patient?

This patient has an endometriotic cyst of her right ovary.

The aetiology of endometriosis is uncertain but three major theories have been advanced. The most popular is that viable endometrial cells spill into the peritoneal cavity during 'retrograde menstruation' and implant on the surface of the pelvic peritoneum and ovaries. An alternative view is that endometriosis may arise from metaplasia of peritoneal endothelial cells anywhere in the abdominal cavity and possibly even the pleural cavities. Lymphatic and vascular spread of endometrium has also been suggested to explain the very rare occurrence of endometriosis in pelvic and inguinal lymphatic glands and other sites. Implantation of endometrium in surgical scars may also occur at the time of hysterotomy and Caesarean section.

Treatment may be either surgical or medical. Surgical therapy is indicated for the removal of ovarian cysts. Enucleation is nearly always possible and sufficient ovarian tissue can usually be left to preserve function. Endometriotic deposits on the peritoneal surface may also be excised or destroyed by diathermy cauterization when found during laparotomy or present in an operation scar. For most women of child-bearing age medial treatment is, however, preferable. This usually involves the oral administration of a combination of oestrogens and progestogens such as ethinyl oestradiol 50 μg and d-norgestrel 250 μg given continuously to suppress ovulation. Atrophy of the endometrial glands and decidual changes in the stroma occur during this treatment which favours necrosis and resorption of the ectopic endometrium. Continuous therapy with high doses of progestogens such as norethisterone 10 mg or dydrogesterone 10 mg twice daily also produces endometrial atrophy and is favoured by some. Somewhat surprisingly cyclical therapy with combined oral contraceptive preparations is also effective despite the withdrawal bleeding it produces. This is probably because very little endometrial proliferation occurs during the treatment-free week. The synthetic steroid, danazol, which suppresses gonadotrophin production, has also been found to be effective for treating this condition.

In women who are over the age of 40 years and have extensive disease, hysterectomy and removal of both ovaries is usually the treatment of choice. This is because removal of the ovaries causes the tumour to undergo spontaneous regression and thus avoids the risk of damage to bowel or other structures which arises when an attempt is made to remove every fragment of endometriosis.

67

A 67 year old man had received treatment for hypertension for ten years and his blood pressure had been moderately well controlled on a diuretic and methyldopa. For two months he had experienced intermittent pain in the lower back which was increasing in severity.

His GP had arranged for X-rays to be taken of his thoracic and lumbar vertebrae, but these had revealed no abnormality.

On the day of admission his pain suddenly increased in severity and was associated with sweating and a feeling of faintness.

On examination, he was distressed and shocked. The pulse was 120/min regular, BP 80/60 mmHg and JVP not visible. The heart sounds were faint and peripheral pulses were present. Examination of the lungs was normal. Inspection of the abdomen revealed faint bluish discolouration of the right loin. Palpation revealed no masses but generalised tenderness was elicited in all areas. Bowel sounds were faint.

1. What is the most likely diagnosis?
2. How may this be confirmed?
3. What urgent therapeutic measures are required?

Low back pain is a common symptom in the middle aged and elderly and has diverse causes. Nevertheless, it is important when presented with such a problem to consider possible causes under certain headings, e.g. skeletal (intervertebral disc, osteoarthritis, Paget's disease, infiltration of bone by malignancy), abdominal (chronic pancreatitis, gynaecological, retroperitoneal tumour), renal or vascular.

The exacerbation of pain associated with shock is a characteristic feature of an aortic aneurysm which has leaked or ruptured. The bluish discolouration of the cutaneous tissues in the right loin indicates the tracking of blood from the site of rupture.

The diagnosis may be made by the finding of a pulsatile mass in the abdomen, associated with an audible bruit, but following rupture and in the presence of shock this may not be palpable.

An X-ray of the abdomen may confirm the diagnosis by demonstrating calcification in the walls of the aneurysmal aorta. (This was indeed present in this case and, in retrospect, was visible on X-rays taken of his lumbar spines one month previously).

The prognosis with rupture of an aortic aneurysm is grave. Immediate transfusion of blood (10-20 units may be required) should be established and arrangements made for major abdominal surgery, where in some cases the aneurysm can be resected and a dacron graft inserted.

68

A 30 year old nursing officer is sent to you because she has been found to have hypertension at a routine examination. She says that her only problem has been headaches which occur almost daily, and that she has had for many years: certainly since she was at school. She had a medical examination when she started nursing school at the age of 18, and was found to be perfectly healthy. She has never been pregnant, and has been taking an oral contraceptive for the last nine years. The lying and standing blood pressures are 210/140 and 200/145 mmHg respectively, and are the same in both arms. The only other abnormal physical sign is narrowed irregular arteries in both optic fundi.

Investigations show —

Serum creatinine 267 μmol/l (normal 62 — 124)

Midstream urine No sugar: moderate protein: 120 WBC per mm^3: no growth on repeated cultures, including T.B. culture.

— and the report on the intravenous pyelogram reads:

'There is no abnormality on the plain film. Both kidneys excrete the dye rather poorly, and injection of a double dose was necessary. The excretion of the dye is symmetrical. The kidneys are regular and smooth in outline, but are both small (10.5 cm from pole to pole) for a patient of this height (1.65 m). The calyces are abnormal: some show diffuse irregularity of their margins, while others extend abnormally into the medulla, sometimes almost cutting off the papilla. The left ureter is dilated and there appears to be a radiolucent object 0.5 x 0.5cm at the lower end of the left ureter. The bladder empties normally.'

1. What is the renal disease: what is the object in the ureter?
2. Could the headaches be relevant?
3. Can she continue to take the oral contraceptive?

The salient features of the renal disease are impaired renal function, showed by the raised serum creatinine and poor function on IVP, a sterile pyuria, small kidneys and abnormal calyces. The calyceal pattern reported is not that of reflux with infection, which would lead to blunted calyces with probably irregular, scarred and shrunken kidneys. Sharp calyces penetrating the medulla, sometimes with irregular margins, are characteristic of analgesic nephropathy. The extension of the calyces is around ischaemic and dying renal papillae, which can become completely separated from the medulla. If papillae that have been sloughed off in this fashion remain in the renal pelvis, they can appear as an island in the urographic dye in the collecting system, so-called 'ring-shadows'. Papillae can also pass down the ureter and may stick at the ureteric orifice or pass *per urethram*. The object in the ureter in this case is probably a renal papilla.

The headaches are not likely to be due to hypertension, as she had them before her medical examination at the age of 18, when she was presumably normotensive. The relevance of her headaches is as a possible reason for analgesic abuse. On further questioning she revealed that she had taken between 12 and 20 analgesic tablets for headaches every day for 12 years, and that until the recent removal of phenacetin from retail sale her usual tablets had been aspirin — phenacetin — codeine mixture. The failure to enquire directly about analgesic use in taking the history was an important omission: all patients who may have renal impairment should be asked about their tablet-taking habits. While analgesic nephropathy is less common in Great Britain than, say, Australia, it is probably more common than is generally realised. It is by no means certain that phenacetin is the only analgesic that can cause renal damage.

Analgesic induced renal failure with hypertension and renal papillary necrosis was probably the sole diagnosis in this patient. However, oral contraceptives can cause arterial disease, and renal ischaemia, with lesions of arteries within the kidneys and hypertension, has been reported in women on the pill. The wise course would be to avoid the risk of further renal damage in a patient who has already suffered considerable loss of kidney function, and to advise a change to a safer form of contraception. This patient found a diaphragm quite satisfactory.

69

An old age pensioner aged 72 consulted her family doctor because of increasing swelling of her ankles and lower legs. One year previously she had been admitted to the local hospital with chest pain and breathlessness, and investigations carried out confirmed the diagnosis of a myocardial infarction. For the past year she had been prescribed digoxin and bendrofluazide and had remained in moderately good health until she became aware of ankle swelling three weeks prior to her consultation. The general practitioner substituted frusemide (40 mg daily) for her bendrofluazide and the limb oedema disappeared. Two weeks later she was admitted as a medical emergency with severe breathlessness and confusion, having 'collapsed' at home.

On admission, she was apyrexial and cyanosed. The pulse was 180/min, irregular; BP 110/70 mmHg. The jugular venous pulse was elevated 6 cm and pitting oedema of the ankles was noted. The heart was enlarged and a systolic murmur was audible on auscultation at the apex. Crepitations were found throughout both lung fields. In the abdomen the liver was palpable 3 cm below the right costal margin and was tender.

1. How do you account for this lady's deterioration?
2. What immediate investigations are indicated?
3. How would you treat this patient?

This lady presents with gross cardiac failure. At this age and particularly in view of her previous history of a myocardial infarct, ischaemic heart disease is undoubtedly present and a recent (silent) infarct may well have precipitated her cardiac failure. At the time of admission she was noted to have an arrhythmia and although possibly associated with a myocardial infarct, one must always consider other causes (e.g. pulmonary embolus). The recent alteration in diuretic therapy, with prescription of a potent diuretic, frusemide, and no potassium supplements, may have led to a state of electrolyte imbalance and hypokalaemia. The latter may precipitate digitalis toxicity and account for her arrhythmia and consequent cardiac failure.

The systolic murmur localised to the apex may merely reflect a dilated mitral valve ring due to gross failure. However, mitral valve dysfunction (ruptured papillary muscle) may occur as a result of a myocardial infarct. (A ruptured intraventricular septum may also complicate a myocardial infarct, give rise to gross cardiac failure, and is associated with the appearance of a systolic murmur).

Immediate investigations must be directed to identifying the nature of the arrhythmia and determining the cause. An e.c.g. therefore is performed and serum electrolytes measured to determine the potassium level. Blood for cardiac enzymes may be taken at the same time in addition to samples for subsequent digoxin estimations. A chest X-ray should be performed.

Electrolyte imbalance must be corrected and, if the serum potassium is low, *gradual* restoration of a normal potassium may be achieved by i.v. infusion. Digoxin therapy should be temporarily discontinued.

The uncontrolled arrhythmia in this patient may be largely responsible for the cardiac failure and attempts should be made to control the cardiac rate. This of course depends upon the electrocardiographic diagnosis of the type of arrhythmia present. However, if a diagnosis of digitalis induced arrhythmia is made, i.v. disopyramide or lignocaine should be given.

70

A 26 year old teacher of American origin was admitted complaining of severe left sided lower abdominal pain and vaginal bleeding. Her last menstrual period had occurred seven weeks before. Her cycle was normally regular with menstruation occurring every 30 days and lasting for seven days but she did occasionally miss a period. She was not using any contraception. Her general health was good and she had been well until two hours before admission when she experienced a severe pain of sudden onset in the left iliac fossa. This was a constant ache with colicky exacerbations. It was worse with movement but did not radiate. Shortly after the onset of the pain she noticed slight vaginal bleeding. She had vomited once and felt faint. There were no micturitional or bowel symptoms, but she had noticed slight breast tenderness. Her past history included a spontaneous abortion six years earlier at 12 weeks pregnancy. She had not had any other pregnancies and was unable to recall any episodes of pelvic infection.

On examination she was anxious, lay very still and was obviously in pain. She was apyrexial and did not appear anaemic. Her pulse rate was 110 beats per minute and blood pressure was 90/70 mmHg. Inspection of her abdomen revealed generally diminished movement with respiration. On examination there was marked tenderness, guarding and rebound tenderness in the region of the left iliac fossa. No mass was palpable and normal bowel sounds were audible. Pelvic examination revealed slight bleeding through the cervix, and marked cervical tenderness with movement. The uterus was difficult to define but appeared to be bulky and anteverted. There was very marked tenderness and resistance in the left vaginal fornix but only slight tenderness on the right side. There was no pelvic mass. Blood was taken for a haemoglobin estimation and white cell count. This showed: Hb 10.5 g/dl, WBC 8.5 x 10⁹/l. A pregnancy test was negative.

1. What was the differential diagnosis?
2. What is the most likely diagnosis and what investigations would you perform to confirm this?
3. Name three aetiological factors.

The most likely diagnosis in this case is a ruptured left tubal ectopic pregnancy. The negative pregnancy test does not exclude the diagnosis as it is only positive in 50 per cent of cases of ectopic pregnancy. Torsion of an ovarian cyst produces a similar clinical picture but the absence of a mass in the case described makes this unlikely. The patient's irregular menstrual cycle also makes it difficult to exclude a ruptured corpus luteum cyst on clinical grounds although the duration of amenorrhoea is more in keeping with a tubal ectopic pregnancy. Unilateral salpingitis is a possibility but is usually associated with a pyrexia and raised white cell count. It is important to realise that it is unusual for a patient with a tubal ectopic pregnancy to display all the classical clinical features such as shoulder tip pain, collapse and gross anaemia. In addition amenorrhoea and even vaginal bleeding may be absent from the history and a palpable mass is usually only present in about one third of cases.

Additional investigation is therefore frequently necessary to confirm the diagnosis before undertaking laparotomy. Of those available laparoscopy is undoubtedly the most valuable.

Aspiration of the pouch of Douglas (culdocentesis) for blood containing small fragments of clot is simpler but is much less reliable. The technique of examination under anaesthesia which relies on the palpation of a tubal mass is negative in as many as 70 per cent of cases and also produces many false positives.

Ectopic pregnancy complicates between one in three to five hundred pregnancies. The most frequent cause is previous pelvic inflammatory disease which may result from acute salpingitis or puerperal or post-abortal infection. Rarely chronic infection such as tuberculous salpingitis may be causative. Other predisposing factors include previous tubal surgery (including sterilisation) and developmental errors of the fallopian tube.

In addition, so called, external migration of the ovum to the opposite fallopian tube may occur when the tube is removed on one side but the corresponding ovary is left *in situ*.

71

A West Indian woman aged 42 had come to England in 1958 and subsequently worked as a packer for a photographic company. She had a son aged 8 years, the product of a normal pregnancy. She had also had a stillbirth of unknown cause.

Four months prior to her attendance at the outpatient clinic her previously normal periods had become heavier and she had experienced lower abdominal pain during the first day of menstruation. Her periods were regular and she had no intermenstrual bleeding, postcoital bleeding, or dyspareunia. Her micturition was normal. She did complain, however, of feeling intermittently faint, and she had occasional 'palpitations'.

On examination she had an 18 week sized mass in the lower abdomen. On bimanual palpation this could not be distinguished from the uterus. Her blood pressure was 170/70 mmHg and auscultation of the heart revealed a systolic flow murmur over the aortic area.

1. What is the most important diagnostic procedure in this case?
2. What haematological investigations are relevant and what would you expect to find?
3. What is the most likely diagnosis?

A definitive diagnosis can only be made by laparotomy. However, routine preoperative investigations such as cervical cytology should not be omitted as they may have an important bearing on the management at the time of operation. Apart from the need to make a diagnosis, even symptomless lower abdominal tumours should be removed if they are larger than 12 weeks size. Laparotomy is therefore an essential part of therapy.

The menorrhagia, faintness, palpitations, wide pulse pressure and aortic flow murmur all suggest an iron deficiency anaemia secondary to chronic blood loss. Investigations (with the results in this case) are therefore:

Haemoglobin	7.5 g/dl
PCV	0.28
MCV	72 fl
MCH	20.4 pg
MCHC	28.7 g/dl
Film	hypochromic
Serum iron	7 μmol/l (normal 14-29)
Iron binding capacity	93 μmol/l (normal 45-72)
Sickle cell haemoglobin electrophoresis	negative

This confirmed the diagnosis and the patient was transfused with three units of packed cells preoperatively.

Both ovarian cysts and fibroids can grow to a large size before they produce symptoms. A complaint of menorrhagia however favours the diagnosis of fibroids. The excessive bleeding is most likely to occur if the fibroids distort and enlarge the endometrial surface, but is also associated with purely intramural growths, possibly due to the resulting uterine hyperaemia. Fibroids are also more common in negresses. It is uncommon for an ovarian cyst to cause anaemia unless it is malignant, in which case other signs such as ascites or an enlarged liver may be present. Parity has a slight effect in that fibroids are more common in nullipara, but as in this case, they also occur frequently in women who have had children.

72

A 60 year old widow was seen by her family practitioner with a complaint of anorexia, weakness, weight loss, shortness of breath and difficulty in swallowing solid foods. She had been well until six weeks previously and led an active life. She stopped smoking (20 cigarettes/day) one month ago because of her dyspnoea and had developed a cough productive of white/grey sputum.

On examination she was centrally cyanosed and dyspnoeic at rest. Fullness of the face and neck were apparent. The radial pulse rate was 100/min, BP 120/80 mmHg; JVP elevated 8 cm; no limb or sacral oedema; the heart sounds were normal. There was dullness to percussion and absent air entry over the right lower zone of the chest and an area of bronchial breathing in the right mid zone. Vocal resonance was absent at the right base. Examination of the abdomen and central nervous system was normal.

A chest X-ray was requested on her presentation to the casualty department.

1. What is the most likely diagnosis?
2. Describe briefly the radiological features you might expect to see on a P.A. chest X-ray.
3. Name three investigations which are likely to confirm your diagnosis.
4. What is the cause of the facial swelling?
5. Outline how you might alleviate the patient's dyspnoea.

The symptoms of anorexia, weight loss and weakness in a patient of this age with chest symptoms suggest a bronchogenic carcinoma or chronic infection. However the nature of the presentation, in particular the associated dysphagia make the former a more probable diagnosis.

The physical signs in the chest are those of a right sided pleural effusion. Thus a dense opacity in the right lower zone possibly associated with shift of the mediastinum to the left would be seen. The presence of dysphagia and superior vena caval obstruction (swollen face and engorged neck veins) indicate a tumour which may be visible as an opacity causing widening of the superior mediastinum.

The diagnosis of a carcinoma of the lung may be confirmed by sputum cytology, bronchoscopy or pleural aspiration and cytology of the pleural fluid. The facial swelling is caused by superior vena caval obstruction.

Dyspnoea is a distressing symptom, and although the tumour is by virtue of its site inoperable, palliative treatment for the relief of the shortness of breath is mandatory. Aspiration of pleural fluid will allow the underlying lung to re-expand temporarily. However, irradiation possibly combined with chemotherapy should be instituted without delay.

This patient had an oat cell carcinoma invading the carina and both main bronchi. Although the SVC obstruction was relieved following irradiation, the patient died ten day later. It was noted that during her admission estimation of plasma sodium was repeatedly low (126 mmol/l) and further studies indicated inappropriate antidiuretic hormone secretion by the tumour.

73

A 22 year old homosexual student presented to the casualty department with difficulty in swallowing. On examination his tonsils were very swollen and inflamed, and he was admitted in case respiratory obstruction developed. On admission, the house surgeon noted a fever (37.4°), and several large, shallow and apparently painless ulcers in the buccal mucosa.

The throat swab that was taken showed no bacterial growth, and the throat surgeon sought the advice of a physician. The only new history elicited was of a 'fissure-in-ano' treated by the patient's general practitioner five weeks earlier, and which had been slow to heal. The physician also found a macular erythematous rash on the face and trunk, and moderate cervical and groin lymphadenopathy.

1. What is the most likely diagnosis? Give one other possibility.
2. List four important investigations.

This history and examination is typical of secondary syphilis. The likely primary lesion was the 'fissure-in-ano'; although chancres are typically painless, a rectal chancre may become painful due to superadded secondary infection, and if at the anal margin this could produce symptoms identical to those of an anal fissure. The skin, pharyngeal and lymph node lesions are usual in syphilis, but an alternative diagnosis would be infectious mononucleosis.

Dark-ground microscopy of exudate from the inflamed tonsils or the mouth ulcers might show spirochaetes, but there is a risk of confusion with saprophytic treponemeta sometimes found in the mouth. Serological tests for syphilis should include specific tests such as examination for fluorescent treponemal antibodies or the treponema pallidum immobilisation test. Nonspecific tests such as the Wasserman reaction may be positive in infectious mononucleosis. Investigations to exclude the latter diagnosis are a full blood count with a differential white cell count (looking for atypical lymphocytes) and tests for heterophile antibody such as the Paul-Bunnell reaction or the monospot test.

The diagnosis of syphilis was confirmed in this patient, and he was treated with penicillin with success. Unfortunately he refused to help in the tracing of his many contacts.

74

A 56 year old widow had been treated by her general practitioner for a mild chest infection. The doctor noted that despite complete resolution of her symptoms of cough and sputum she remained unwell and extremely lethargic. For some months she had complained of loss of weight (0.5 kg) and vague abdominal pains that were unrelated to food.

No abnormal signs were found on examination of her chest but the G.P. referred the patient to hospital for further investigation.

In the outpatient clinic the following observations were made: general weakness, areas of white depigmented skin on the forearms, pulse 80/min regular, BP 90/60 mmHg. The heart and lungs were clinically normal and no abnormalities were discovered on examination of the abdomen or central nervous system.

Investigations revealed: Hb 13.1 g/dl; WBC 6 x 10⁹/l; plasma sodium 126 mmol/l; potassium 5.0 mmol/l; urea 15 mmol/l. Chest X-ray normal.

1. What is the most likely cause of this patient's presentation?
2. What other clinical features might have been present?
3. Give two conditions which may be associated with this condition.
4. Suggest two investigations for confirmation of the diagnosis.

Hypotension, vitiligo and hyponatraemia in a middle aged person who gives a history of weight loss, abdominal pain and lethargy suggest a diagnosis of Addison's disease. A sudden exacerbation in symptoms may be precipitated by an intercurrent illness such as the chest infection in this case. In this age group an underlying malignancy should also be considered.

One of the characteristic features of Addison's disease is pigmentation which, although not invariably present, must be looked for with particular emphasis on the mucus membranes of the mouth and the palmar creases. 'Idiopathic' or autoimmune adrenocortical atrophy is the most common form of this disease but bilateral involvement of the adrenals by tuberculosis or malignant disease can rarely occur, in which case symptoms and signs of the primary disease may be found.

Addison's disease may be associated with other organ specific autoimmune diseases such as pernicious anaemia and myxoedema. Diabetes mellitus is a rare associate.

The most important investigations are those of determinations of plasma cortisol. Samples should be taken at midnight and early morning (06:00) to confirm the low levels encountered in Addison's disease.

Adrenal failure may be consequent upon a pituitary lesion, thus differentiation of primary and secondary Addison's disease may be determined by measurement of cortisols following ACTH stimulation.

75

A 26 year old Spanish woman who was married to a waiter was pregnant for the third time. Her first two pregnancies, three and four years before in Spain, had both ended in spontaneous mid-trimester abortions (at 17 and 14 weeks). In the present pregnancy she attended the antenatal clinic for the first time at 12 weeks when bimanual palpation confirmed that the uterine size was compatible with her dates. A careful examination of the cervix, performed because of her past obstetric history, however, revealed a short (one centimetre long) cervical canal which easily admitted a finger. A diagnosis of cervical incompetence was made and a Shirodkar suture was inserted two days later under general anaesthesia. At each of her subsequent fortnightly visits to the clinic a vaginal examination was performed to ensure that the cervix remained closed.

Her pregnancy progressed uneventfully until thirty two weeks when she was admitted to the labour ward as an emergency complaining of severe lower abdominal pain. On examination she was apyrexial but appeared shocked and anaemic with a blood pressure of 75/50 mmHg and a pulse rate of 124 beats per minute. Abdominal palpation revealed a uterus of 36 weeks size which was tense and tender. It was not possible to determine the fetal lie or presenting part with certainty and the fetal heart could not be heard either on direct auscultation or using a doppler ultrasonic heart detector. A mid-stream urine specimen was obtained which was found to contain one 'plus' of protein and ketones on testing with dip sticks.

1. Give a differential diagnosis and indicate which is the most likely?
2. How would you manage this patient?
3. What complications may occur as a result of this condition?

This patient has suffered a concealed accidental antepartum haemorrhage (*abruptio placentae*). The localisation of the tenderness to the uterus and its tenseness help to exclude other causes of an acute abdomen in pregnancy, such as torsion of an ovarian cyst, intestinal obstruction, acute pyelonephritis and appendicitis. The absence of fetal heart sounds reduces the likelihood of other uterine causes such as acute hydramnios and red degeneration of a fibroid. Advanced extra-uterine pregnancy and uterine rupture are possibilities but are excessively rare.

The principles underlying treatment are 1) correction of shock by blood transfusion and pain relief 2) when this has been achieved to empty the uterus and 3) to prevent complications.

These patients display shock which appears to be out of proportion to the intrauterine bleeding. Blood must therefore be taken for haemoglobin estimation, cross matching of fresh whole blood (at least four pints) and plasma fibrinogen estimation. An intravenous infusion through a wide bore cannula should be set up and freeze dried plasma administered while awaiting blood. The foot of the bed should be raised and an intramuscular injection of morphine (15 mg) given immediately.

Estimation of intrauterine blood loss is impossible and a central venous pressure line (CVP) should be inserted and enough fresh whole blood transfused to restore the CVP to 10 cms of water. If only packed cells are available then one unit of reconstituted freeze dried plasma should be given with each unit of packed cells. Between 2 and 5 g of fibrinogen should also be administered.

As soon as the shock is corrected a vaginal examination should be performed, the Shirodkar suture removed, and the membranes ruptured. Labour usually follows rapidly but if the uterus is not contracting actively within an hour an oxytocin infusion should be commenced.

An indwelling Foley catheter must be introduced into the bladder and careful monitoring of urine output maintained (oliguria or anuria may occur due to renal failure following the severe hypotension). Release of thromboplastins into the general circulation from the retroplacental clot may provoke disseminated intravascular coagulation and lead to a hypofibrinogenaemic coagulopathy. This is why fresh whole blood is so vital in these patients. Should the patient's blood fail to clot or her plasma fibrinogen fall below 100 mg/dl, additional fibrinogen (5-10 g) must be given and labour should not be induced until the coagulation disorder has been corrected.

These patients also display an increased incidence of post partum haemorrhage and 0.5 mg intravenous ergometrine should be given with the delivery of the stillborn baby.

76

A 23 year old girl was brought into casualty having admitted to taking 80 assorted tablets containing aspirin and paracetamol two hours previously. She complained of ringing in her ears and said that she had vomited on one occasion.

On examination she was fully conscious and orientated. Pulse 100/min, BP 110/70 mmHg. Heart normal. The respiratory rate was 40/min, but the remainder of the examination was normal.

1. What is the mechanism underlying her overbreathing and what metabolic abnormalities may occur in this situation?
2. Outline your urgent management of this case.

Two days later she appeared to have recovered uneventfully and took her own discharge from hospital. On the fifth day, however, she began to feel ill and returned to hospital.

3. Why did she return to hospital?

Respiratory stimulation occurs in the early stages following a large dose of salicylates and this accounts for the girl's hyperventilation. As a consequence a respiratory alkalosis develops, but the acid-base status is complicated by a metabolic acidosis produced by several factors which include the uncoupling of oxidative phosphorylation, salicylic acid itself and in severe cases renal insufficiency.

Delayed gastric emptying may occur with salicylate overdose and a gastric washout is indicated in this situation as unabsorbed aspirin may be removed from the stomach.

Blood samples must be obtained initially for salicylate and paracetamol levels, and repeated two hours later. The purpose of the second sample is to determine whether or not the plasma level of drug is increasing. With elevated levels of salicylate ($>$ 700 μg/ml four hours after ingestion) a forced alkaline diuresis is indicated to facilitate the urinary excretion of the ionised fraction of the drug. Forced diuresis does not promote paracetamol excretion.

With a conscious patient careful observations must be recorded at frequent intervals of respiratory rate and amplitude of breathing, pulse rate and blood pressure. If respiration is impaired, ventilation must be assisted by respirator. The circulatory state if depressed requires intravenous infusions to maintain central venous pressure and an adequate cardiac output. Fluid replacement must be carefully monitored and in all cases measurements of blood ureas and electrolytes performed together with assessment of urine flow for evidence of renal impairment.

Paracetamol levels if high ($>$ 300 μg/ml, four hours after ingestion) give rise to hepatocellular damage and recent evidence suggests this may be prevented by the administration of cysteamine or methionine.

The return of the girl to hospital five days following her overdose could well be due to the development of jaundice as a consequence of paracetamol induced liver damage. This complication is frequently not apparent in the first few days after taking the overdose.

77

Two patients presented with a lump in the neck.

The first was a Malaysian Chinese student aged 24, who had lived in England for 3 years. The lump was in the left side of his neck, just above the clavicle: it had gradually enlarged over the preceding eight weeks. He had generally otherwise been well, although on one or two occasions he had awoken at night bathed in sweat, and his skin felt itchy. Six years previously he had had a similar but smaller lump removed from the other side of his neck. On examination, the scar from this operation could be seen in the right anterior triangle. The new lump was in the left anterior triangle, arising from behind the clavicle. It was 6 cm wide and 2 cm from front to back: the surface of the mass was not fixed to the skin and felt lobulated, and the consistency was firm and rubbery. The mass seemed fixed to deeper structures.

The second patient was a man of West Indian origin. He was 30 years old and had lived in London for ten years. There was no past history of note. The lump was on the right side of his neck, under the ear: he had suddenly noticed it four days previously, but his wife said she had seen it three weeks before. He had been more concerned about pain and weakness in his right arm that had got progressively worse over the last four weeks. He had lost some weight, and had suffered night sweating attacks. Examination showed a firm fixed tender mass 3 cm by 2 cm behind the right sternomastoid, with weakness and wasting of the muscles of the right arm supplied by C7, and an absent triceps jerk.

1. Give at least three possible diagnoses that would fit either case.
2. What is the one investigation that would be most likely to establish the diagnosis in either case?

The lumps in both cases, from their description, almost certainly arose from lymph nodes, and the problem is that of the differential diagnosis of chronically enlarged cervical lymph nodes.

Chronic lymphadenopathy is likely to be due to chronic infection or to infiltration with neoplasm. The lymphadenopathy of infectious mononucleosis, secondary syphilis, or toxoplasmosis is transient rather than persistent and progressive. Lymphadenopathy secondary to a pyogenic infection elsewhere could present as in these cases, except that the nodes would be very tender and would not tend to mat together as in the first case: also the site of the primary infection should have been found on examination. The chronic infection that is most likely, especially in those born abroad, is tuberculosis. The past history in the first case is a little suggestive of tuberculosis, with previous excision of a lump that may have been a tuberculous node. Both cases have had night sweats, typical of a tubercular infection.

Possible neoplasms are many. Primary neoplasms of lymphoid tissue include lymphatic leukaemia, lymphosarcoma and reticulum cell sarcoma. In this age group these are all less common than Hodgkin's disease. Hodgkin's disease often starts in cervical nodes, and they typically feel rubbery, as in the first case, who also shows fever and pruritus, common systemic manifestations of Hodgkin's disease. The second case, with fever and weight loss, could also have Hodgkin's disease, with the additional problem of a deep seated mass of Hodgkin's tissue compressing the seventh cervical nerve root. Both cases could also have a secondary neoplasm growing in their nodes, with a primary carcinoma elsewhere. This is perhaps the most likely diagnosis in the second case, as carcinoma is more prone to invade and compress neural tissue than is primary neoplastic lymphoid tissue or a simple inflammatory or tuberculous mass.

The one investigation likely to give a definite diagnosis in either case is biopsy of an affected node. This was performed. The diagnosis in the first case was nodular sclerosing Hodgkin's disease; and in the second, rather unexpectedly, was tuberculosis.

78

On a Sunday evening you are called to see a 37 year old man in casualty who has presented with a one week history of intermittent fever and sweats. He is anorexic and feels unwell with headache, a dry cough and generalised aches and pains. Two weeks previously he had returned from a business trip to Kenya.

On examination he was obviously ill with a pyrexia of 39°C and a few slightly elevated red spots were present on the chest. Examination of the cardiovascular system revealed pulse 90/min regular, BP 100/70 mmHg, JVP not elevated and heart normal. The chest was clear; there was slight abdominal tenderness and the spleen was just palpable.

Investigations carried out in the casualty department were as follows: Hb 12g/dl; WBC 3 x 10^9/l; blood urea and electrolytes normal; chest X-ray normal.

1. How would you manage this patient?
2. Give three diagnoses and appropriate investigations.
3. What is the treatment of your most probable diagnosis?

The man has a febrile illness which follows a visit to Africa. The cause must be presumed to be infective and he should be isolated immediately until the diagnosis has been established. This may be arranged in an isolation ward or by transfer to a hospital for infectious diseases.

This illness has many suggestive signs and symptoms of typhoid fever — fever, abdominal discomfort, bronchitis, splenomegaly and 'rose-spots' (note that diarrhoea is not always an accompaniment of this disease). However many other infectious diseases present with similar features and must be considered, e.g. malaria, tuberculosis, brucellosis and certain viral (e.g. influenza) and rickettsial diseases. The presence of rose-spots in this patient make the diagnosis of typhoid fever most probable.

An attempt should be made to isolate the organism and in this case cultures of blood, stool, urine and rose-spots should be obtained. Increased titres of the O & H antigens of *S. typhi* (Widal test) are found by the third week of the illness.

If a diagnosis of typhoid is not substantiated by investigation, further tests should include a thick blood smear for malarial parasites; Mantoux test and bone marrow aspiration and culture for tubercle together with culture of sputum (if present), gastric aspirate, urine and stool for acid fast bacilli. In brucellosis agglutinins may be identified in high titre in serum. Rickettsial disease is characterised by a positive Weil-Felix agglutination test.

Chloramphenicol is the drug of choice in the treatment of typhoid fever and the drug should be prescribed for a period of two weeks (50 mg/kg/day). Ampicillin (4 grams/day) is also effective.

Contacts must be identified and immunized.

79

A 22 year old married comptometer operator presented in her first pregnancy after 11 weeks of amenorrhoea. She was 151 cm tall and weighed 50 kg. The pregnancy progressed normally and she was admitted at 38 weeks gestation in established labour. Abdominal examination revealed a longitudinal lie, cephalic presentation, with the head unengaged. The cervix was 3 cm dilated but uneffaced and firm. Artificial rupture of the membranes was performed and fetal monitoring commenced. Uterine activity was assessed via an intrauterine catheter and was normal.

Four hours later the contractions were still normal and the cervix was 4 cm dilated. However, after a further four hours the contractions became less intense and a vaginal examination showed the cervix to be unchanged. An intravenous infusion of oxytocin was commenced and increased steadily up to 12 mU/min. which improved her contractions but twelve hours after the initial examination she was still only 4 cm dilated. The cervix was not well applied to the head which was in the occipito-transverse position. There was a considerable degree of caput formation although the head was still unengaged in the pelvis. The degree of moulding was difficult to determine because of the extent of the caput.

1. What is the most likely cause of this patient's slow progress in labour?
2. What is the likely outcome?
3. What postpartum investigation would you like to perform?

The commonest cause of slow progress in labour is inadequate uterine activity. This can be demonstrated by measurement of intrauterine pressure. It is corrected by oxytocin infusion and normal progress will then ensue unless there is an additional factor, as there clearly was in this case. Other causes of arrested progress which are important because they are remediable are a full bladder or rectum. An unfavourable cervix will produce a prolonged labour because of the lengthened latent phase but assessment of the 'ripening' of the cervix (by means of the Bishop score) will reveal that progress is in fact taking place. Pelvic masses (such as fibroids) or an enlarged fetal head (hydrocephalus) can also cause labour to become obstructed, but these should normally be detected in the antenatal period. This leaves the possibility of cephalopelvic disproportion due to a small pelvis. This is made all the more likely by the patient's small stature, and the failure of the head to engage in the pelvis throughout labour.

The complete arrest of progress over eight hours in this case despite normal uterine activity makes it most unlikely that a vaginal delivery could have been achieved. The outcome was therefore a lower segment Caesarean section. A live male infant weighing 3.3 kg was delivered in good condition. Postpartum pelvimetry should be performed to determine management in the next pregnancy. The measurements in this case were: A.P. inlet 10 cm, midcavity 11 cm, outlet 10 cm, transverse inlet 11 cm, interspinous 9.5 cm intertuberous 11.5 cm. Antepartum pelvimetry is usually only performed when absolute cephalopelvic disproportion is suspected. This is because even with accurate ultrasound measurement of the fetal head it is impossible to predict the outcome, as the degree of moulding which will occur in labour cannot be known in advance. Careful assessment of the progress of labour, ensuring that there is adequate uterine activity, and close attention to the condition of the fetus is now the preferred management.

80

The patient was a 65 year old export manager. She was a childless widow, and lived alone: she had formerly smoked and drank heavily (her husband had been in the colonial service), but for the last five years she had drunk alcohol only at Christmas and smoked less than 5 cigarettes each day. She was left handed and was taking no drugs.

Her presenting complaint was of numbness in the left hand. This had been gradual in onset, starting with the ulnar border of the hand, and over about one week spreading to involve the whole hand. She had noticed some clumsiness in the movements of her left hand, which progressed over about 4 weeks so that she had difficulty in fastening buttons or picking up a pencil with her left hand. This clumsiness was more marked if she did not look at the object she was trying to manipulate. Her symptoms then remained stable for 6 weeks, until she awoke one morning with a large area of numbness involving part of the left forearm: she thought that the clumsiness of the left hand was also more marked.

General physical examination showed locomotor brachialis, rather hard radial arteries, and absent pulses in the right leg below the femoral pulse. There was a bruit over the right femoral pulse, but no other bruits were heard. Apart from generally rather brisk reflexes, abnormal neurological signs were confined to the left hand. There was no weakness or wasting, and the tone was normal. Pain, temperature and vibration sensation were normal, but there was slight subjective impairment of light touch over the whole of the left hand, and joint position sense was not perfect. Two-point discrimination was markedly impaired in the left hand, and she could not identify a key or a pen placed in that hand if she had her eyes closed. Coarse movements were well coordinated, but fine 'piano-playing' movements of the fingers of the left hand were clumsy, and she appeared to have genuine difficulty in fastening buttons with this hand.

1. Where is the neurological lesion?
2. What is a likely cause of the lesion?

The neurological symptoms and signs in this case are mostly sensory. They are not in the distribution of a particular peripheral nerve, nor can they be attributed to one or other of the main sensory tracts in the spinal cord. Impaired two-point discrimination and astereognosis (inability to recognise objects by touch alone) are predominant features, and these are associated with lesions of sensory areas of the cerebral cortex. Astereognosis suggests a lesion of the contralateral (right, in this case) sensory parietal cortex, just posterior to the main sensory cortex in the posterior central gyrus. Such a lesion affects fine sensory discrimination, with impaired subjective response to light touch, and produces disordered perception of the position of the affected part in space, thus explaining the abnormal joint position sense and the awkwardness in making fine movements.

As usual when making a neurological diagnosis, the disordered function shows the site of the lesion, but not the pathology: the time-course of development of the symptoms and signs is the clue to the underlying disease. Steadily worsening symptoms and signs suggest a neoplasm or other steadily growing space occupying lesion, and this would be the presumptive diagnosis after the first 4 weeks of this patient's illness. However, the sudden exacerbation of symptoms 6 weeks later suggests a vascular event (haemorrhage, thrombosis or embolism). The general examination in this case gives evidence of widespread atherosclerosis, and therefore vascular lesions of the brain are likely: the brisk reflexes suggest that there is diffuse upper motor neurone ischaemia. Neoplastic and vascular disease can coexist: for example, the late exacerbation in this case could be due to a small haemorrhage into a tumour.

A further complication: rarely, repeated small emboli going to one area of the brain can produce a progressively worsening ischaemia at that site and thereby mimic the progressive behaviour of a neoplasm. That is what happened in this patient. She was investigated in the days before computerised axial tomography, so the most important tests were isotope brain scanning, air encephalography and carotid arteriography.

The first two were normal, and the latter showed no abnormality apart from stenosis and marked irregularity of the right internal carotid artery in the carotid siphon in the base of the skull. It was thought that this was the source of repeated emboli.

81

A 75 year old lady had been in a remarkably good state of health for her age until three months prior to her consultation with the family doctor. She complained of feeling tired, but the reason which had precipitated her visit to the surgery was a complaint of pain beneath the right breast and in the right side of the chest wall. The pain had come on gradually, at first being a minor discomfort but latterly a continuous 'nagging pain'. Two days prior to her consultation a rash had appeared at the site of the pain.

On examination, although well preserved for her age, she was pale. Palpable lymph nodes were evident in both axillae and the supraclavicular fossae. A vasicular rash was present in the 5th right intercostal space radiating round the trunk to the spine. In the abdomen, the liver was just palpable, but no other masses were found. Examination of the cardiovascular, respiratory and central nervous systems were normal.

Preliminary investigations revealed:— Hb 9.5 g/dl WBC 83 x 10⁹/l, of which lymphocytes were 75 x 10⁹/l. The platelet count was 100 x 10⁹/l.

1. What is the diagnosis and how do you account for the reduced haemoglobin?
2. What is the most likely cause of this patient's rash?
3. Outline your treatment?
   1. Of her haematological disease.
   2. Of the cutaneous lesion.

The blood count in this case reveals moderate anaemia and thrombocytopenia with a gross elevation in the white cell count, most of these cells being mature lymphocytes. These haematological features are characteristic of chronic lymphatic leukaemia and the diagnosis is further substantiated by the clinical findings of axillary and supraclavicular lymphadenopathy.

The anaemia of chronic lymphatic leukaemia is usually normochromic and normocytic and may result from impaired erythropoeisis, increased red cell breakdown or from haemorrhage. However, a Coombs positive haemolytic anaemia may be present.

The painful vesicular rash present in this patient has a characteristic dermatome distribution and was caused by herpes zoster. Note that immunosuppression is a common problem in patients with leukaemia and various infections may intervene in the course of the illness.

The asymptomatic patient with chronic lymphatic leukaemia may have treatment withheld since many such patients have a disease which runs a relatively 'benign' course. This patient, however, is both anaemic and thrombocytopenic and appropriate chemotherapy should be instigated. Chlorambucil or corticosteroids or both may be effective in inducing remission. Radioactive phosphorous is an alternative therapy.

Transfusions may be required for anaemia and haemorrhage. Scrupulous attention must be paid to the early diagnosis of infections and appropriate measures taken to treat these.

Topical applications of idoxuridine in dimethylsulphoxide may partially relieve the pain of herpes zoster and may accelerate healing. Oral analgesics, e.g. aspirin, paracetamol, are also useful. However, if severe herpetic pain is present and persists despite the use of more potent analgesics, local nerve blocks with phenol will provide relief of pain.

82

A 23 year old laboratory technician presented in the accident and emergency department with a three day history of swelling of the right labium majus, which had become acutely painful over the previous 24 hours. She was otherwise well. She said she had never had sexual intercourse and on examination she was indeed virgo intacta. There was a red, swollen, fluctuant mass in the lower half of the right labium majus but no vaginal discharge. She was afebrile.

She was admitted and the mass was incised under general anaesthetic. The incision was made just inside the vagina over the point of maximum tension. A large amount of foul smelling pus was evacuated. Adhesions within the cavity of the abscess were broken down digitally and the incision marsupialized. Swabs were sent for culture.

1. What was the aetiology of the abscess?
2. What would be likely to grow on culture of the swabs?
3. What antibiotics should be prescribed?

A Bartholin's cyst starts as a retention cyst of one of the Bartholin's glands. A minor skin inflammation (such as that produced by wearing tight clothes with inadequate ventilation) is on occasion sufficient to block the ducts of the gland. Secretions build up behind the blockage and form a cyst. Such a cyst is liable to become infected at any time.

As in this case, there is often no growth unless the swab is collected in a medium suitable for anaerobic organisms (such as Robertson's cooked meat). This is because common infecting organisms are gram negative anaerobic bacilli, which are normally bowel commensals. (They are also a common cause of wound infection following abdominal surgery). The organism can also be a skin commensal such as *Staphylococcus aureus*, or other bowel organisms such as *Escherischia coli*, *Streptococcus faecalis*, or Proteus. In a woman with an active sexual life, the gonococcus should be also considered, and swabs taken into Stewart's transport medium for immediate culture. (*Neisseria gonorrhoeae* is a very fragile organism outside the genital tract and will not survive for very long without optimal conditions of temperature and carbon dioxide concentration).

Antibiotics are not usually required in the treatment of an incised Bartholin's abscess. Proper drainage plus thrice daily salt baths almost invariably results in prompt resolution. Pain is cured immediately by incision and relief of tension in the gland. The inflammation settles rapidly over the next three to four days, and at ten days the incision will be hardly visible. In the rare event of an inflammation persisting, an antibiotic should be chosen according to the results of the culture. It will commonly be ampicillin supplemented by metronidazole for the gram negative anaerobes.

83

A 34 year old woman was pregnant for the first time. For three years she had been treated for mild hypertension by her family practitioner and at the time of her first visit to the antenatal clinic, her blood pressure was 150/90 mmHg and she was taking hydrochlorothiazide (25 mg daily). The drug was changed to alphamethyldopa on which her blood pressure was well controlled until 32 weeks gestation when the pressure rose to 180/110 mmHg and she developed oedema.

She was admitted to hospital and hydralazine was added to the treatment which temporarily controlled the pressure but she went into premature labour.

An intravenous salbutamol infusion was set up in an attempt to suppress uterine contractions. Shortly thereafter she developed acute pulmonary oedema.

1. How do you account for the development of pulmonary oedema?
2. What important physical sign should have been recorded?
3. What therapeutic error was made?

It is probable that the precipitation of left ventricular failure in this woman was a result of the intravenous infusion of salbutamol and might have been avoided if the pulse rate had been recorded prior to the infusion. Reference to the patient's charts showed that the heart rate was 120/min at this time and rose rapidly with the salbutamol.

A number of factors were undoubtedly contributory to the onset of pulmonary oedema. The blood pressure reduction that occurs with the vasodilator drug hydralazine is accompanied by a reflexly mediated rise in heart rate, in addition to salt and water retention. Infusing a drug which, despite its claimed selectivity for ß2 receptors undoubtedly has an effect on the heart, would have an additive effect and lead to a progressive rise in heart rate.

Contributory factors resulting in the development of heart failure include the high output state characteristic of late pregnancy, the increased circulatory blood volume and the obvious fluid retention.

In this case, the high pulse rate should have alerted the obstetrician to the potential hazard that could be encountered with a ß stimulant drug and salbutamol should not have been given.

Alphamethyldopa has been implicated in this drug interaction, although the mechanism remains obscure.

84

Mrs X's medical troubles began in childhood. She had bilateral mastoidectomies, a tonsillectomy, bronchopneumonia and scarlet fever, all by the age of twelve years. She had a dilatation and curettage for frequent heavy periods at the age of twenty, followed by two normal pregnancies. Following the birth of her children she took the contraceptive pill but complained of severe headaches and nausea and so was changed to the intrauterine contraceptive device. This caused very heavy and painful periods so that at the age of thirty six the coil was removed. The heavy periods continued and so a total hysterectomy with conservation of the ovaries was performed. At the age of thirty eight she presented complaining of frequency and urgency so that sometimes she wet herself. She also had nocturia, needing to pass urine eight times each night. Examination at this time showed a normal vagina with a well supported anterior wall. An intravenous pyelogram, urine culture and cystoscopy were all normal. She was sent for a videocystogram which was reported as follows:

'There was catheter discomfort. The bladder held 510 ml. The supine cystomyogram was normal, but the erect filling caused a small contraction at the end. On coughing, the neck opened and the pressure rose. The flow rate was 30 ml per second at a normal pressure of 35 cm of water but there was a high kick to 55 cm on stopping. This bladder is unstable on erect filling and there is a cough trigger'.

1. What type of bladder disorder does this patient have?
2. What surgical and medical approaches are there to treatment?
3. What is the long term prognosis?

In the diagnosis of urinary incontinence in the female it is extremely important to distinguish between stress incontinence and urge incontinence. This is because the treatment of the two conditions is so different. The former is associated with loss of the urethrovesical angle (sometimes due to prolapse) while the latter is due to the much more difficult problem of detrusor irritability.

Stress incontinence is characterised by an involuntary and unheralded loss of urine on straining. It is usually abolished by lying down, and hence nocturia is not a major problem. Urgency on the other hand usually produces an intense desire to micturate before any urine actually appears. The patient described therefore has urgency incontinence. The condition is often associated with other psychosomatic complaints and the patient's very full medical history is typical. However, disseminated sclerosis or any other neurological abnormality should always be excluded by careful examination before a label of 'psychosomatic' is appended.

The initial treatment was with the anticholinergic drugs epronium bromide and amitriptyline hydrochloride, the latter of which is also an antidepressive. This was not completely successful. An attempt at bladder retraining was therefore made in which the patient was admitted to hospital and required to hold her urine for set periods of time, starting with ten minutes and increasing daily. This regime succeeded in producing a significant improvement in her complaints.

Because of the difficulty of treatments such as bladder retraining, and the tendency of many patients to relapse and require further courses of treatment, there is a great temptation in cases of urge incontinence to attempt a surgical correction. This is almost always a dismal failure, and the temptation should be strongly resisted.

85

A 75 year old woman is sent to hospital because her general practitioner is worried about her renal function. The lady has been healthy, apart from a tendency to intractable urine infections, until about six months previously, when she developed mild ankle oedema. The general practitioner gave her hydrochlorothiazide 50 mg and amiloride 5 mg each day, starting six weeks before admission, and this cleared the oedema. One week before admission she complained of thirst, and was noted to be drowsy. On the day before admission plasma sodium was 129 mmol/l, potassium 6.1 mmol/l and urea 62 mmol/l (normal 2.5-6.6 mmol/l).

On examination, she is drowsy and is dehydrated, with reduced skin turgor and eyeball tension. There are no other abnormal physical signs of note. She has a catheter in her bladder, which is draining small volumes of foul smelling urine resembling thin pus. Investigations on admission show: plasma creatinine 279 μmol/l (normal 62-124 μmol/l); chest X-ray — slight aortic unfolding, normal lung fields; plain X-ray of the abdomen — kidneys of normal size, with bilateral staghorn calculi.

1. What may be the cause of her impaired renal function?
2. Why is the plasma urea proportionately more abnormal than the plasma creatinine?
3. If she is to be rehydrated by intravenous infusion, which fluid would you give?
4. What would be the general principles of treatment of her presumed urinary infection?

There are two possible causes for the renal impairment in this lady, and one cannot decide which came first. The primary problem may be a tendency to renal stone formation, with consequent obstruction to urine flow and secondary infection in the structurally and functionally deranged urinary tract: or, the first abnormality may have been recurrent infections, which can (especially if the organisms are urea-splitting), predispose to urolithiasis. Whether the renal failure is due to an obstructive uropathy or to chronic bacterial pyelonephritis, the principles of initial treatment are the same.

The relatively mild elevation in plasma creatinine concentration shows that renal damage is not very severe. Plasma urea is affected by the protein content of the diet and by the state of hydration much more than is the plasma creatinine, and the results in this patient, together with the physical signs, show that she has moderate renal impairment which has been exacerbated by dehydration. There are two reasons for the dehydration. The first is her renal disease: conditions such as obstructive renal failure or chronic pyelonephritis, which attack the tubules rather than the glomeruli, lead to impaired urine concentrating power with a tendency to waste sodium and water. This problem has been exacerbated by the prescription for diuretics, which has promoted even more marked loss of salt and water.

The correct initial treatment is therefore rehydration with 'normal' (0.9 per cent) sodium chloride solution. A common error is to give sodium-poor fluids, such as 5 per cent dextrose or 'dextrose-saline'. These make the problem worse by diluting further the already abnormally low plasma sodium.

Urine must be sent for culture, but attempts to eliminate all infection might be injudicious and probably ineffective. The likely findings on culture would be a mixture of organisms, mostly resistant to the usual antibiotics. Once the patient has been rehydrated, and urine flow is again reasonably brisk, it is unlikely that there will be any symptoms that would be relieved by treating the infection. The most that should be attempted is treatment of any new infecting organism that causes new symptoms (for example, dysuria), and local measures to improve bladder hygiene — this includes removal of the catheter as soon as is reasonably possible.

86

A 36 year old nurse complained of weakness, lassitude and headaches, and was found to be hypertensive. She was admitted to hospital for investigation. The only other symptom that she mentioned to the house physician was abdominal pain, which had previously been shown by barium meal examination to be due to a gastric ulcer. She took a variety of medicines for her ulcer, some bought at the chemist and some stolen from the drug trolley on her ward. She smoked more than 30 cigarettes each day, and said that she drank wine. She was not taking an oral contraceptive, and had never been pregnant. On examination her blood pressure was 160/120 both lying and standing. She was obese and there was slight epigastric tenderness, but physical examination was otherwise normal.

The initial investigations showed:

Hb	11.2 g/dl
MCV	108 fl
Plasma sodium	138 mmol/l
potassium	2.8 mmol/l
bicarbonate	31 mmol/l
Urine sodium	46 mmol/24 h
potassium	60 mmol/24 h
Plasma renin activity	180 pmol/l/h (normal 400–1800)

1. Could the abnormalities in these results be related to her symptoms or to her hypertension?

After one week in hospital, before any treatment had been prescribed, her blood pressure was 150/100 and repeat investigations showed:

Plasma sodium	137 mmol/l
potassium	4.2 mmol/l
bicarbonate	27 mmol/l
Urine sodium	218 mmol/24 h
potassium	42 mmol/24 h

2. Suggest a possible cause for the changes in urinary and plasma electrolytes.
3. Give two reasons why the blood pressure may have fallen.

The haematological abnormality in the first set of results is a mild anaemia with large red cells. Macrocytic anaemias are due to deficiency of vitamin B_{12} or of folate, and while there may be many causes for such deficiencies, there are clues in the history in this case. The patient drinks wine in unspecified quantities, and excess alcohol can cause macrocytosis by interfering with folate metabolism. The gastric ulcer may be related to the abnormal haematology in two ways: gastric ulcers are more common in those who abuse alcohol (as well as in smokers), and blood loss from the ulcer may have contributed to the anaemia. If the patient is indeed a heavy drinker, this may have some relation to her hypertension: there is epidemiological evidence linking excess alcohol consumption with high blood pressure.

The initial electrolyte abnormality is an hypokalaemic alkalosis with an inappropriately high renal excretion of potassium and a reversal of the usual urine sodium/potassium ratio. This suggests that a sodium retaining, potassium losing agent is present in this patient, i.e. a mineralocorticoid or mineralocorticoid-like substance. Mineralocorticoid excess can be primary, or secondary to a high plasma renin which is stimulating aldosterone release from the adrenal cortex. The low renin in this case shows that the mineralocorticoid excess is primary: either an adrenal adenoma secreting aldosterone (Conn's syndrome), adrenal hyperplasia, excess cortisol (which has some mineralocorticoid activity), or an exogenous agent taken by the patient. These electrolyte changes are possibly connected both with her symptoms — weakness and lassitude are usual in hypokalaemia from any cause, and are common in Conn's syndrome — and, through sodium retention, with her hypertension.

The electrolyte changes have completely resolved a week after admission to hospital. The electrolyte picture in Conn's syndrome is not necessarily constant, but complete reversal to normal would be unusual. A more reasonable explanation is that the mineralocorticoid activity was in a substance that the patient was taking, but stopped on admission. As she has helped herself to drugs from the trolley, it is possible that she has taken carbenoxolone (which has strong mineralocorticoid activity) for her ulcer. Another salt-retaining substance she could have taken, and obtained more innocently, is liquorice.

One reason for the fall in blood pressure may be this withdrawal of salt-retaining substances. However, an important alternative reason is the spontaneous fall in blood pressure usually seen after rest in hospital. Remember that high blood pressures tend to improve to some extent without drugs when assessing the response of hypertensive patients to treatment.

87

A 27 year old dancer, married to a musician, had commenced regular intercourse at the age of fifteen. She had a number of sexual partners but never used any contraception, and became pregnant at the age of twenty. She had a normal delivery at thirty four weeks gestation of a male infant which was subsequently adopted. She then used the oral contraceptive 'pill' and continued with this after her marriage two years later. She obtained supplies at six monthly intervals from her general practitioner and all went well until she missed two consecutive withdrawal bleeds. Alarmed lest she had become pregnant, she attended a family planning clinic. A routine cervical smear was taken which showed markedly dyskariotic cells with mitotic figures present suggesting a carcinoma *in situ*.

1. What factors in the history suggest the need for regular screening of cervical cytology?
2. What investigation will help to delineate the extent of the lesion?
3. What is the treatment?

The exact aetiology of carcinoma of the cervix is unknown but there is a strong association with sexual intercourse. In particular, the risk is highest in those who commence coitus at an early age and those who have multiple partners. This latter fact suggests the possibility of a slow virus infection; in general the wider the exposure the more likely the infection. Thus, no cases of cervical carcinoma were discovered in a study of the death certificates of 13,000 nuns. Regular screening should however be carried out in all women who indulge in regular sexual activity, but particularly if, as in the case described, they have had multiple partners. Unfortunately, those at risk are often the least likely to attend a clinic regularly. A request for contraception therefore provides a good opportunity to take a cervical smear.

The most widely used investigation is the cervical cone biopsy (or conisation). This involves removing a cone shaped portion of the cervix so that a precise histological diagnosis can be made. This will show whether the malignant cells are entirely confined to the epithelium (stage 0, carcinoma *in situ*, intraepithelial carcinoma), microinvasive (stage 1a, invasion less than five millimetres), occult invasive carcinoma (invasion more than five millimetres but not clinically apparent, still stage 1a) or invasive (stage 1b, so long as the carcinoma is confined to the cervix). The affected area can be delineated before removal with the use of Lugol's iodine (Schiller's test) in which the malignant cells (which do not contain glycogen) remain white while the normal vaginal epithelium stains brown-black.

A more precise delineation which will also give some information as to the severity of the lesion is colposcopy. This involves examination of the cervix with a low power binocular microscope (x 8). It is particularly useful in pregnancy if the patient does not wish to have it terminated, since, provided the lesion is not invasive, it is possible to be reassured that there is no immediate danger, and defer treatment until after delivery (conisation during pregnancy is associated with an increased risk of bleeding and abortion). Indeed, when the patient is re-examined eight weeks after delivery, in about fifty per cent the lesion is found to have regressed and surgery is not necessary.

The patient described proved not to be pregnant, and colposcopy showed the lesion to be of no more than average extent. In particular the lesion did not extend up the cervical canal, indicating that the cone need not be taken too deeply (a very deep cone carried the subsequent risk of cervical incompetence or fibrotic stenosis). For a carcinoma *in situ* or microinvasive carcinoma the cone biopsy itself is intended to be curative (which explains why it is often called conisation rather than 'biopsy'). For this reason it is important to delineate the affected area carefully to avoid leaving behind any malignant tissue. After conisation, the woman should be followed up with regular smears for the rest of her life (or at least until the age of sixty years). If histology unfortunately shows that the malignant tissue has invaded more than five mm, the treatment of choice is Wertheim's hysterectomy, radiotherapy, or both.

88

The senior registrar arranged immediate admission for a patient he saw in the clinic. She was a young mother who was prone to develop allergic rashes on antibiotics which she took for recurrent cystitis and urethritis. Two days earlier she had started on a course of co-trimoxazole, which she had taken once before with no trouble. 24 hours before the clinic visit her face and jaw had begun to swell, she noticed difficulty swallowing solid food, and her breathing became stertorous. She was indeed greatly swollen about the lower part of the face, and her throat could not be examined because of the swelling, which was painful.

The senior registrar diagnosed angio-oedema, and gave subcutaneous adrenaline, antihistamines, and steroids. When the patient arrived in the ward, 30 minutes later, she was no better. The house physician made the correct diagnosis, and she confirmed it by taking blood for amylase, which was 2,400 U/1 (normal less than 300).

1.   What is the correct diagnosis?

This is mumps. The senior registrar made two mistakes. The first was to assume that disease in a patient prone to allergy was likely to have an allergic cause. This made him forget a common problem and think of a rarity. Angio-oedema (sometimes still called angioneurotic oedema) is due to a defect in the mechanisms of complement, and could present as a drug reaction in the manner described, with the exception that the swelling would probably not be painful — the second mistake.

A young mother would be likely to come into contact with many small children, and so would be especially prone to catch their viruses. A raised amylase is common in mumps, and may be of pancreatic or of salivary origin.

89

An English typist became pregnant at the age of nineteen. She had never used contraception despite regular intercourse for four years, and only discovered she was pregnant after eighteen weeks of amenorrhoea. As she was single and wishing to pursue her career, she had a termination of pregnancy performed by instillation of urea and prostaglandin into the amniotic fluid.

She married at the age of twenty two and soon became pregnant, only to miscarry at twenty weeks gestation. Her next pregnancy, a year later, ended the same way. In her fourth pregnancy, a cervical suture was inserted at fourteen weeks. She remained in hospital for three days and then went home. At thirty weeks the membranes ruptured spontaneously and she was readmitted to hospital. The rupture of the membranes was confirmed by speculum examination. The cervical suture was still in place, there was no bleeding and the cervix appeared to be closed. Fetal presentation was cephalic and there was no evidence of uterine contractions.

1. What was the probable cause of her obstetric problems?
2. What are the hazards facing the fetus?
3. Outline the management which you would adopt.

This patient's initial problem was recurrent midtrimester abortion, associated with cervical incompetence, probably produced by trauma to the cervix at the time of termination of her first pregnancy. Vaginal termination before twelve weeks of amenorrhoea is unlikely to damage the cervix but forcible dilatation to the size of an eighteen week fetus can produce disruption of cervical tissue with subsequent competence of the internal os. The diagnosis can sometimes be confirmed in the non-pregnant state by the gentle passage of cervical dilators of increasing size until resistance is felt, or by an X-ray cervicogram using radio-opaque dye to outline the cervix. In the current pregnancy, the cervix had been held closed by a suture. However, once the membranes have ruptured, the suture acts as a septic focus for ascending infection of the amniotic fluid. This can produce a severe endometritis and septicaemia in the mother and can produce an intrauterine pneumonia in the fetus.

Endometritis will stimulate uterine contractions, producing premature delivery with the risk of respiratory distress due to pulmonary immaturity. Infection may also cause fetal distress in labour. The priority in management is therefore to remove the cervical suture. The patient should be given a parenteral broad spectrum antibiotic, such as ampicillin or a cephalosporin, which will cross the placenta. Dexamethasone, 4 mg three times daily, may be given orally or intramuscularly in an attempt to reduce the risk of the infant developing hyaline membrane disease (respiratory distress due to pulmonary immaturity). This is maximally effective after 24-48 hours, and therefore if contractions occur, they should be supressed for at least this length of time with an intravenous infusion of a sympathomimetic drug such as ritodrine or salbutamol. However, if the patient develops a pyrexia or other signs of infection, labour should be allowed to progress, since the dangers of infection are the most serious. Once the dexamethasone has been given for 48 hours, the patient should be delivered by stimulating labour with an oxytocin infusion, since prolonged rupture of the membranes may lead to infection with an antibiotic resistant organism.

Careful monitoring of the fetus should be performed during labour, preferably by cardiotocography and fetal blood sampling where necessary. Caesarean section should be performed urgently if there is any sign of fetal distress. There is an increased risk of intracranial haemorrhage at birth in preterm infants, and a generous episiotomy with careful control of delivery of the head is therefore important. If the presentation is by the breech, an elective Caesarean section should be performed because the risk of damage to the aftercoming head becomes unacceptably high.

90

A 73 year old chronic bronchitic man was transferred to a medical ward for further investigations and management following an operation for the removal of a cataract in his right eye. His operation had proceeded uneventfully and there had been no post-operative chest complications of his anaesthetic.

He had had a similar operation on his left eye three months previously which had been successful.

Seven days after his recent operation he lost his appetite and felt generally unwell. He was noted to be jaundiced by the house officer and urinalysis showed urobilinogen and bilirubin to be present in excess. His liver was enlarged and tender on palpation.

Relevant investigations were as follows: Hb 12 g/dl; WBC 6 x 10⁹/l; platelets normal; blood urea and electrolytes normal; aspartate aminotransferase 495 iu (5-30); bilirubin 170 umol/l (5-17); alkaline phosphatase 162 iu (20-95); plasma proteins normal.

1. How do you account for the development of jaundice?
2. What further investigations would you perform?

This elderly man has hepatocellular jaundice, characterised by the markedly raised transaminase and bilirubin with only moderate elevation of the alkaline phosphatase. The temporal relationship between the onset of jaundice and the recent operative procedure suggests a causal link and halothane jaundice was considered a probable diagnosis when it had been established that this anaesthetic gas had been used during both operations. A detailed history was obtained, but no other drugs known to cause hepatocellular jaundice had been taken, (methyldopa, rifampicin, isoniazid, etc.).

One cannot rule out the possibility that the jaundice was due to a viral infection such as viral hepatitis and a history of recent contacts should be sought. Furthermore, the identification of possible sources of hepatitis ß would be appropriate (history of blood transfusions, etc.) and Australia antigen should be determined in a serum sample.

Halothane hepatitis is uncommon, considering the vast number of operations carried out in which halothane is used as an anaesthetic gas. It is more likely to occur when two or more anaesthetics are administered within six months of each other. Re-exposure to halothane in patients who have recovered from halothane jaundice will cause a recurrence of the jaundice.

Repeated assessment of liver function must be carried out as the condition may progress to massive hepatic necrosis and death. Where the diagnosis is in doubt and if liver function deteriorates liver biopsy should be performed after ensuring that prothrombin time and platelet counts are normal.

91

A 40 year old publican was drunk by closing time every night. He would be abusive and uncoordinated, and his wife therefore left him well alone until the morning. One night he fell down the cellar stairs, landing head-first on the stone floor. His wife found him lying there in a pool of vomit the next morning. He was able to tell her what had happened, but when he arrived in the casualty department one hour later he was deeply unconscious and not responding to pain. The casualty officer noted that the left pupil was normal, but that the right pupil was widely dilated and made no response to light, although light shone in the right eye made the left pupil contract.

1. What operation is needed at once?
2. What is the other emergency that presents with an ophthalmoplegia in alcoholics? It is not associated with injury: a typical patient with this syndrome might be ataxic and drowsy, with a poor memory, and have nystagmus in addition to weakness or paralysis of external ocular movements. The pupils might be normal or abnormal.

The history of deepening unconsciousness a few hours after injury, with development of an unilateral opthalmoplegia, is typical of acute intracranial bleeding into the extradural or subdural space. The opthalmoplegia is usually but not invariably on the side of the bleeding, and is due to indirect pressure on the third cranial nerve. The optic nerve is not affected, as shown by the normal consensual light reaction of the left pupil. The diagnosis is easy in a young patient with a clear history of injury, but can be difficult in the elderly, in whom the injury necessary to cause intracranial bleeding may be very slight indeed. The correct treatment in this case is immediate burr hole exploration of the skull, beginning on the side of the dilated pupil.

Wernicke's encephalopathy is the syndrome described in the second question. It is seen in alcoholics, often those with a demonstrably deficient diet. The essential features are ophthalmoplegia (which often includes palsies of conjugate gaze and lateral rectus weakness), nystagmus, and ataxia. There is often drowsiness and listlessness, which may progress to coma and death. There may be a failure of short term memory, with confabulation (Korsakoff's psychosis) and some patients show a peripheral neuropathy or cardiac failure in addition. Wernicke's syndrome is a medical emergency, as it may progress rapidly if the correct treatment — large doses of thiamine — is not given. The prognosis for the ophthalmoplegia and ataxia in the treated case is excellent: the improvement in Korsakoff's psychosis with thiamine treatment is usually only slight.

92

A thirty five year old Jordanian teacher booked at fourteen weeks in her seventh pregnancy. She had no significant medical history but her father was a diabetic taking oral hypoglycaemic drugs and her mother was being treated for hypertension.

Her past obstetric history was as follows:

1962   a term female, weighing 3.5 kg. No complications.

1963   a term male, weighing 3.5 kg. No complications.

1964   a term male, weighing 3.0 kg. The patient became anaemic antenatally, and required a blood transfusion after delivery.

1965   a term female, weighing 3.5 kg. The patient had a post partum haemorrhage, necessitating a blood transfusion.

1967   a term male infant, weighing 4.0 kg. No complications.

1972   a term male infant, weighing 4.6 kg. The patient had a postpartum haemorrhage, necessitating a blood transfusion.

1.   What obstetric grouping does this patient fall into?
2.   List the complications for which this group is at increased risk.
3.   What special precautions would you take to anticipate them?

This patient is a grand multipara. The definition of this group is variable but the term is normally applied to women who have had four or five previous viable babies.

The complications most likely to occur are anaemia, both in the antenatal and postpartum period, placental abruption, malpresentations (due to a lax abdominal wall), precipitate labour, fetal macrosomia (which can obstruct labour, producing uterine rupture), and postpartum haemorrhage. In addition, the grand multipara is often in an older age group, with a raised perinatal mortality rate due to hypertension or placental insufficiency or both.

Care must be taken to ensure an adequate diet and supplements of iron and folic acid should be given. A social worker may need to help with arrangements to ensure that the patient gets enough rest during the pregnancy.

If the patient lives any distance from the hospital, admission at 39 weeks gestation is often necessary to avoid the baby being born on the journey in. Elective induction at term in favourable cases may also be employed, particularly if the lie of the fetus is unstable. Postpartum haemorrhage is a real and serious threat, and the patient should have at least two pints of blood crossmatched as soon as she goes into labour.

Intravenous ergometrine at delivery (in the absence of hypertension) is useful prophylaxis against haemorrhage, and one must be prepared to perform a manual removal of the placenta without undue delay if it fails to separate readily.

Careful monitoring of fetal growth in the antenatal period with serial oestrogen or human placental lactogen estimations and biparietal diameter measurement is indicated if the patient is over thirty or hypertensive. Fetal monitoring in labour is also important.

This patient has two potential diabetic features in her history, namely, diabetes in a first degree relative and a previous infant that weighed more than 4.5 kg at birth. It would therefore be wise to perform a glucose tolerance test at 28 weeks to detect possible gestational diabetes.

93

A soldier aged 19 was on manoeuvres. He was lying on his back in long grass when a motor-cycle dispatch rider accidentally drove over his upper abdomen from right to left.

On arrival in casualty 40 minutes later he was conscious and breathing spontaneously, although sweating and in great pain. There were superficial abrasions on the right side of his trunk at the level of the 10th and 11th ribs. The chest was normal on examination although he was breathing rapidly. The pulse rate was 130 and the blood pressure 85/40 mmHg. The abdomen did not move on respiration, and on palpation it was exquisitely tender, and rigid all over. No bowel sounds could be heard. Power and sensation in the legs were normal.

1. Which two therapeutic measures are essential?
2. Are any investigations that help with the diagnosis needed?

The immediate questions that must be asked about any victim of major trauma are: is the airway clear? — is respiration adequate? — is the circulation in danger? There is no immediate danger to the airway or to respiration in this patient, but he is shocked. There is peritoneal irritation, and the likely diagnosis is shock due to intra-abdominal bleeding from a ruptured spleen, ruptured liver, or torn mesentery: there may also be damage to other intra-abdominal structures. He appears to have avoided injury to the spinal cord, although there is always the risk that an unstable fracture of the spinal column will cause delayed trauma to the cord. The pelvis is well away from the site of the injury, so damage to the pelvic viscera is unlikely.

The therapeutic measures needed are to restore blood volume, and to stop the bleeding. Each of these is useless without the other. An intravenous infusion through a large bore cannula must be started at once, using saline or a plasma expander until blood is available. A laparotomy must be arranged as soon as possible. Restoring the blood volume, and finding and controlling the bleeding, are essential to save life. However, the therapy that the patient would probably feel was most important is relief of pain. Analgesia should be adequate, but safe — depressing neither respiration nor blood pressure.

This patient had a ruptured liver. He needed 40 units of blood before and during surgery. Haemostasis was secured following hemihepatectomy.

A 28 year old man complained of painful, tender swellings on his shins. Two weeks previously he had had a sore throat associated with 'flu-like' symptoms and had been given penicillin by his family doctor. On further questioning he admitted to having lost 4 kg in weight during the past three months. In addition, he had a cough productive of little sputum and had, on two occasions, coughed up a small amount of blood.

On examination, the only abnormal physical signs were the presence of several 1-3 cm diameter, raised, red, tender lumps on the anterior surface of both lower legs.

Preliminary investigations revealed: Hb 12 g/dl, WBC 6 x 10⁹/l, ESR 90 mm/h.

i. What is the most likely skin lesion present in this case?
2. Give three aetiological factors which should be considered.
3. What further investigations would you perform?

The description and distribution of the skin lesions in this case is characteristic of erythema nodosum. (Some insect bites, however, may look remarkably similar). This condition may be associated with a number of unrelated disorders, several of which are possible in this patient.

An untoward drug reaction should always be considered as a cause of a cutaneous eruption, and in the case of erythema nodosum, penicillin, sulphonamides, sulphonylureas and oral contraceptives have all been implicated as causative agents. In addition, ß-haemolytic streptococcal infections may be associated with this condition and it is possible that the throat infection which occurred two weeks before the onset of the rash was due to this organism.

The history of weight loss, cough and haemoptysis extending over a period of three months suggest a more chronic illness such as tuberculosis. Both tubercle and sarcoid are associated with erythema nodosum.

Important investigations include a throat swab and sputum examination for acid fast bacilli and culture. A raised antistreptolysin titre would indicate a recent streptococcal infection and a chest X-ray must be performed.

The Mantoux (1 in 10 000) was strongly positive in this case and apical consolidation was present on the chest X-ray; sputum grew tubercle bacilli.

95

An English housewife presented at the age of 25 years with 12 weeks of amenorrhoea in her first pregnancy. She was sure of her dates. Her blood pressure at booking was 120/80 mmHg. Her urine was sterile and showed no protein on dipstick testing. She had no history of renal disease. Examination confirmed the stage of gestation.

Her pregnancy progressed normally until 35 weeks gestation when her blood pressure rose to 150/95 mmHg. She was admitted for rest and observation. Serial ultrasound cephalometry was commenced, as was twice weekly 24 hour urine collection for oestrogen excretion estimation. Daily fetal cardiotocography was performed. All these tests were normal and her blood pressure fell to normal within two days of admission. After five days in hospital she was allowed home, with instructions to rest as much as possible. She was seen weekly at the antenatal clinic.

Antenatal investigations continued to be normal, with evidence of good fetal growth, until four days before term when her blood pressure rose again, this time to 160/105 mmHg. Her urine showed ++protein on dipstick testing. She was admitted directly from the clinic. Over the next 24 hours her hypertension was maintained, and an Esbach test showed a proteinuria of 3 gms per 24 hours. Cardiotocography showed a normal fetal heart rate with a reactive pattern. Vaginal examination showed the cervix to be long, hard and closed with a Bishop score of one.

1. What condition did this patient have?
2. What is the main risk in this situation?
3. Which clinical feature is most worrying?
4. Outline your management.

This patient had pregnancy associated hypertension, otherwise known as toxaemia of pregnancy or pre-eclamptic toxaemia. The aetiology of this condition is unknown. The mild form in which there is hypertension alone (variously defined as greater than 140/90 mmHg or a diastolic pressure greater than 20 mmHg above the booking pressure) occurs in 10 per cent of patients. It is most common in first, multiple and diabetic pregnancies. It tends to occur towards term and may represent an exaggerated physiological response to failing placental function as the placenta ages. It does not usually carry an increased risk for the fetus as the normal results of fetal monitoring in this case testify. The main danger is that the condition may become fulminating, with the risk of eclampsia (fits), which does carry a high fetal mortality and even a maternal mortality (eclamptic fits are still the third most common cause of maternal death in this country). Fulminating pre-eclampsia occurs in only about 1.5 per cent of all patients, or about 15 per cent of those with mild pre-eclampsia. The most reliable indication that pre-eclampsia is becoming fulminating is the appearance of proteinuria (greater than 500 mg per 24 hours). Once this appears, perinatal mortality is increased three fold. Oedema alone is no longer considered a significant clinical feature.

The only effective treatment of fulminating pre-eclampsia is termination of the pregnancy, since the risk of fits becomes very small after 24 hours of the puerperium, and negligible after a week. In most cases the proteinuria disappears shortly after delivery and blood pressure returns to normal within six weeks. While delivery is being arranged, an anti-convulsant may be administered to protect against fits. If the hypertension becomes severe, hypotensive agents such as hydralazine are used to reduce the risk of cerebrovascular accidents.

Induction of labour can be difficult with a very unripe cervix. In this case the cervix was dilated by the insertion of a Foley's catheter filled with 30 ml of sterile water and left in place for 12 hours, and partially ripened by the local application of prostaglandin E2. Labour was then induced by artificial rupture of the membranes and intravenous oxytocin infusion. After 11 hours a healthy male infant weighing 3.4 kg was delivered vaginally. If the labour had progressed slower than expected, or the blood pressure gone out of control, Caesarean section would have been performed.

96

A 47 year old woman arrived in England by plane from Los Angeles. She was staying at a London hotel and consulted a doctor because of a complaint of frequency of micturition and dysuria for which she was prescribed an antibiotic.

Four months previously she had had a hysterectomy for fibroids and her post-operative recovery had been complicated by a deep venous thrombosis of the right calf. Since that time she had been prescribed anticoagulants which she took regularly.

One week after her first consultation with the hotel doctor for urinary infection she awoke in the night with a severe pain in the right side of her chest. The pain was severe, sharp in character and exacerbated by breathing. She also complained of breathlessness and was observed to be sweating profusely.

She was transferred to hospital where on admission she was noted to be extremely dyspnoeic and cyanosed. The pulse rate was 110/min, sinus rhythm; BP 100/70 mmHg; JVP raised 5 cm. The heart was not clinically enlarged but on auscultation the second heart sound was prominent in the second left intercostal space. There were no abnormalities on examination of the lungs or abdomen.

1. Give the cause of this women's chest pain.
2. What may have precipitated this presentation?
3. Outline your immediate management of this case.
4. Should her condition deteriorate what action would you take?

The sudden onset of pleuritic pain associated with dyspnoea, cyanosis and evidence of right heart strain is highly suggestive of a pulmonary embolus, particularly in view of the previous history of a deep venous thrombosis.

Relative immobilisation during travel such as occurs during a long flight may predispose to venous thrombosis. This was a likely precipitating factor in this case. Note that antibiotics may potentiate the action of oral anticoagulants due to a reduction in vitamin K synthesis by gut flora — this contrasts with the reduction of anticoagulant effects observed for example when drugs with enzyme inducing properties are administered, e.g. barbiturates.

This woman shows signs of cardiac strain resulting from a grossly compromised pulmonary circulation. Oxygen must be administered immediately and the extent of oxygen desaturation of the blood determined from arterial blood gas analysis. A chest X-ray and e.c.g. should be perfomed. The former may reveal signs of pulmonary infarction. However, in the early stages radiological abnormalities may be difficult to detect. In gross cases areas of decreased vascular markings may be evident. A ventilation-perfusion isotope lung scan may be useful in diagnosis.

It is necessary to determine the efficiency of her existing anticoagulant therapy by measurement of the prothrombin time. However, with this presentation substitution of oral anticoagulants with intravenous heparin is indicated.

Pain should be relieved with appropriate analgesia. If opiates are necessary, careful monitoring of lung function by repeat blood gas analysis is mandatory.

If her condition deteriorates pulmonary angiography will delineate the extent of pulmonary arterial occlusion. Therapy with a fibrinolytic agent such as streptokinase may be instituted, but if there is no improvement pulmonary embolectomy must be considered after consultation with a cardiothoracic surgeon.

97

A 58 year old housewife had noticed a vulval lump of increasing size for two years. This had caused local soreness and was associated with a low abdominal 'dragging' sensation. Menstruation had ceased eleven years earlier but for the past three months she had been troubled by an intermittent blood stained vaginal discharge. She had not had intercourse for some months because of the discomfort which it caused.

On vulval inspection there were moderate atrophic changes and when the patient was asked to bear down the cervix became visible at the introitus. Its surface was ulcerated. When she stood up the vaginal walls became everted. Palpation of the resulting prolapse revealed that the entire uterus was lying outside the vulva.

1. What is the diagnosis?
2. What other symptoms may occur in this condition?
3. What factors predispose to utero-vaginal prolapse?
4. What treatment would you recommend?

The patient has a third degree prolapse or complete procidentia, with decubital ulceration. This type of prolapse is inevitably associated with a large cystocoele and the patient may have difficulty in emptying her bladder completely. Some residual urine is often present and this may cause diurnal frequency of micturition. Chronic cystitis may follow with frequency during the day and night together with urgency and dysuria. In those cases where there is bladder prolapse without descent of the urethra, the patient may also have difficulty in starting to pass urine unless she first pushes up the base of the protruding bladder. A large rectocoele may produce a similar difficulty with defaecation and the patient may find it necessary to push the rectocoele back before she can empty her bowels.

The precise aetiology of genital prolapse is uncertain but atrophy of the uterine ligamentous supports due to oestrogen deficiency arising after the menopause is undoubtedly an important factor. This appears to unmask a pre-existing weakness which may be congenital or acquired. It is generally stated that trauma sustained during childbirth is a major predisposing factor as less than five per cent of women who develop prolapse are nulliparous. Genital prolapse is, however, uncommon before middle age and as the majority of women (at least 80 per cent) in this age group are parous the association between childbearing and prolapse does not necessarily indicate a causal relationship. On the other hand it is possible that in some women a difficult vaginal delivery may exacerbate a prior weakness leading to a prolapse in later life.

Another factor which may precipitate a prolapse in susceptible women is increased intra-abdominal pressure e.g. due to chronic cough, abdominal tumour formation, ascites or chronic constipation.

A ring pessary should be fitted to this patient to ensure that the ulcer heals, and infection should be eradicated using local chemotherapy. When this has been achieved a vaginal hysterectomy with an anterior and a posterior repair should be performed. For lesser degrees of prolapse the Manchester operation with a posterior repair is usually the treatment of choice unless there are uterine symptoms which themselves warrant hysterectomy.

98

A 22 year old clerk who was fit and healthy with no previous medical history was walking home from his office when he experienced a sudden sharp and severe pain on the right side of his chest. The pain increased in severity and he became short of breath and had to rest on a park bench. He took a taxi to his doctor's surgery from which he was referred to the local casualty department. Six months previously he admitted to a similar experience but on that occasion the pain was on the left side of his chest and although exacerbated by breathing was not accompanied by any significant dyspnoea.

On admission he denied a cough, was apyrexial, but slightly breathless. Abnormal physical signs were confined to the chest.

1. What is the most likely diagnosis?
2. Describe the abnormal physical signs you might expect to elicit in the chest.

During the time he spent in the casualty department, he became progressively dyspnoeic.

3. What physical signs and radiological features would be important to elicit?
4. Outline your management of this case.

The abrupt onset of pleuritic chest pain associated with dyspnoea in an otherwise fit young man is highly suggestive of a pneumothorax. The similar episode six months previously adds support to this diagnosis, as pneumothoraces are frequently recurrent. The absence of a previous history of a respiratory infection and apyrexia makes an infective cause of pleurisy unlikely. Pleuritic pain associated with a pulmonary embolus should always be considered but, although not ruled out by the negative history and lack of evidence for a peripheral venous thrombosis, it is not a probable diagnosis in this case.

The physical signs elicited from this patient with a pneumothorax included diminished expansion of the right chest, a hyperresonant percussion note over the right side of the chest, reduced tactile vocal fremitus and vocal resonance and reduced or absent air entry on the affected side.

Deviation of the trachea to the left and shift of the mediastinum to the left both clinically and radiologically signify the development of a tension pneumothorax. The chest X-ray will also reveal the absence of lung markings on the right side, and the urgent therapeutic procedure is the insertion of an intercostal tube to permit the release of the air under pressure through an underwater-seal bottle.

In less severe cases without 'tension', it is reasonable to wait for two or three days to see whether the lung will re-expand on its own, but failing this a similar procedure to that described for a tension pneumothorax should be adopted.

Patients should be fully informed of the problem, since more than half are likely to experience a subsequent pneumothorax.

99

A 56 year old lady complained of a headache and difficulty with vision. The headache came on suddenly at night. It was constant, very severe, bilateral, and extended from the frontal region to the occiput. Soon after the headache began she vomited, and this made the pain worse. She noticed that her vision was abnormal the next morning: she tended to see double, and to see properly she had to keep her left eye closed. Her husband noticed that the left eye seemed a little turned out, and that the eyelid was drooping.

Her doctor, who had been treating her with a diuretic for hypertension, advised her that it was probably a virus, but she felt no better the next day. At this stage she tried to walk but her back was painful and she could not bend down to pick anything up. Because her son was a doctor she telephoned him at his work, and he made the correct diagnosis from the above history.

1. What is the most likely diagnosis?
2. Suggest the most important investigation in establishing this diagnosis, and the most important investigation in planning the definitive treatment.

Headache arising from intracranial structures is usually due to pathological changes in blood vessels or in the meninges. The sudden onset of headache in this case suggests a vascular event, but the distribution of pain over the whole head, and later extension to the back with inability to bend down, suggests meningeal pain. Putting these two features together, the likely diagnosis is a subarachnoid haemorrhage, probably from an intracranial arterial aneurysm, occurring suddenly at night, with blood spreading over the intracranial subarachnoid space, and then tracking down the spinal subarachnoid space with neck and back pain and stiffness. Patients with severe headache of any cause can vomit, and the vomiting can make the pain feel worse: in this case there was probably further bleeding with the rise in blood pressure that occurs with vomiting. There are two other features in the history that would fit our diagnosis. The first is the pre-existing hypertension, which is common in patients with subarachnoid haemorrhage. The second is the eye signs.

The combination of ptosis and an abducted eyeball is due to a third cranial nerve lesion, with involvement of the nerve fibres to levator palpebrae superioris, and unapposed action of the sixth cranial nerve. The lesion is not complete or else the ptosis would be severe enough completely to obscure the pupil, so that the patient could not detect her own strabismus by suffering diplopia. Acute third nerve lesions can be due to diabetes mellitus, thiamine deficiency, meningovascular syphilis and often intracranial aneurysm of the circle of Willis. The third nerve is closely related anatomically to the circle of Willis, so an expanding or bleeding aneurysm can easily impinge on the nerve.

The diagnosis of subarachnoid haemorrhage can be confirmed, provided that there is no papilloedema, by lumbar puncture. If this is done soon after the bleed, the cerebrospinal fluid will be uniformly bloodstained. In time, the red cells will lyse, and the fluid becomes xanthochromic.

If an intracranial aneurysm has bled once it is likely to bleed again, and surgery to attempt to prevent this is probably beneficial. The site of the aneurysm must be known before operation, so cerebral angiography must be performed. The optimum time for this to be done is a matter of debate, but is probably a few days or a week after the haemorrhage when the patient is in a more stable state than immediately after the bleed. The radiologist would start with the left carotid artery in this case, as the aneurysm is likely to be on that side: if none were seen, the right carotid and then the vertebrals would be examined.

100

The patient was a 78 year old man, who had been coming to the outpatient clinic for some time. He had cardiac failure, which was controlled on digoxin and diuretics, the doses of which had been adjusted from time to time over the years. At one visit the dose of digoxin was increased to 0.125 mg daily: the diuretic treatment was hydrochlorothiazide 25 mg daily. He was taking no other drugs.

When he was seen by the consultant in outpatients at the next visit he gave a history of nausea for 4 weeks, constipation for 3 weeks, and increasing shortness of breath for 1 week. On examination, the pulse rate varied between 40/min (regular) and 130/min (irregular), and the patient was in cardiac failure that was worse than it had been for some years.

He was admitted to hospital at once.

1. What is the likely cause of the new symptoms and signs?
2. Suggest at least 2 investigations that must be done on the night of admission.
3. Outline the immediate treatment.

The combination of gastrointestinal symptoms and cardiac arrhythmias, with failure of control of cardiac decompensation in this patient is almost pathognomonic of digoxin toxicity, and this must be the working diagnosis. The dose is very small, but the elderly are particularly sensitive to digoxin.

The two investigations that are most urgent are an electrocardiogram and measurement of the plasma electrolytes and urea. The e.c.g. will show the nature of the arrhythmias, and also the characteristic e.c.g. effects of digoxin (notably the prolonged P-R interval and the sagging S-T segments: these by themselves do not constitute toxic effects and may be seen when the dose is in the therapeutic range). The arrhythmias in this patient are likely to include episodes of complete heart block and episodes of tachyarrhythmia of ventricular, nodal or atrial origin, all of which are found in digoxin poisoning. Digoxin is particularly dangerous if the plasma potassium is low, and if there is renal failure. A low plasma potassium is particularly likely in a patient taking a thiazide without a second, potassium retaining, diuretic, or without effective potassium supplementation. A high plasma urea in this patient might suggest that there is some renal impairment, but it is important to remember that diuretics can induce a reversible rise in blood urea in the absence of renal failure.

A chest X-ray would be useful to assess the degree of cardiac failure, particularly in comparison with earlier or later films. Plasma digoxin levels are of little value in such a case, as there is a range of plasma digoxin within which some patients are well controlled and others are showing symptoms and signs of toxicity.

The immediate treatment is to stop digoxin, control cardiac failure, and ensure that no harm results from the arrhythmias. The cardiac failure should be controlled with diuretics, taking care to keep the plasma potassium within the normal range using potassium retaining diuretics and potassium supplements as appropriate. Continuous monitoring of the e.c.g. would be a wise precaution, and dangerous arrhythmias — for example, those causing a marked fall in cardiac output or those known to be likely to precede cardiac arrest — should be treated. In particular, complete heart block may need transvenous pacing.

Index

This index classifies the case histories in three ways. The first section is by 'speciality', although such divisions may be arbitrary, and may overlap: many cases appear under more than one heading. The next section is 'presentation', and is an index of the main presenting symptoms and signs of each case. The last section is 'diagnosis'. In many of the obstetric cases the problem is one of management rather than of diagnosis, and the entries under 'presentation' and 'diagnosis' are the same.

N.B. The index refers to CASE numbers only *not* pages.

N.B. The index refers to CASE numbers only *not* pages.

N.B. The index refers to CASE numbers only *not* pages.

N.B. The index refers to CASE numbers only *not* pages.